What You Need to Know about Diabetes

**Recent Titles in
Inside Diseases and Disorders**

What You Need to Know about Autism
Christopher M. Cumo

What You Need to Know about ADHD
Victor B. Stolberg

What You Need to Know about ALS
Harry LeVine III

What You Need to Know about Eating Disorders
Jessica Bartley and Melissa Streno

What You Need to Know about Diabetes

Tish Davidson

Inside Diseases and Disorders

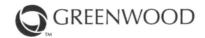

An Imprint of ABC-CLIO, LLC

Santa Barbara, California • Denver, Colorado

Library of Congress Cataloging-in-Publication Data

Names: Davidson, Tish, author.
Title: What you need to know about diabetes / Tish Davidson.
Description: Santa Barbara, California : Greenwood, an imprint of ABC-CLIO, [2020] | Series: Inside diseases and disorders | Includes bibliographical references and index.
Identifiers: LCCN 2019059989 (print) | LCCN 2019059990 (ebook) | ISBN 9781440868603 (hardcover) | ISBN 9781440868610 (ebook)
Subjects: LCSH: Diabetes. | Diabetes—Treatment. | Diabetics—Family relationships.
Classification: LCC RC660 .D375 2020 (print) | LCC RC660 (ebook) | DDC 616.4/62—dc23
LC record available at https://lccn.loc.gov/2019059989
LC ebook record available at https://lccn.loc.gov/2019059990

ISBN: 978-1-4408-6860-3 (print)
       978-1-4408-6861-0 (ebook)

24 23 22 21 20   2 3 4 5

This book is also available as an eBook.

Greenwood
An Imprint of ABC-CLIO, LLC

ABC-CLIO, LLC
147 Castilian Drive
Santa Barbara, California 93117
www.abc-clio.com

This book is printed on acid-free paper ∞

Manufactured in the United States of America

This book discusses treatments (including types of medication), diagnostic tests for various symptoms, and organizations. The authors have made every effort to present accurate and up-to-date information. However, the information in this book is not intended to recommend or endorse particular treatments or organizations, or substitute for the care or medical advice of a qualified health professional, or used to alter any medical therapy without a medical doctor's advice. Specific situations may require specific therapeutic approaches not included in this book. For those reasons, we recommend that readers follow the advice of qualified health care professionals directly involved in their care. Readers who suspect they may have specific medical problems should consult a physician about any suggestions made in this book.

For Helen and Susan

Contents

Series Foreword ix

Acknowledgments xi

Introduction xiii

Essential Questions xv

CHAPTER 1
What Is Diabetes? *1*

CHAPTER 2
The History of Diabetes *13*

CHAPTER 3
Causes and Risk Factors *31*

CHAPTER 4
Signs and Symptoms *41*

CHAPTER 5
Diagnosis, Treatment, and Management *45*

CHAPTER 6
Long-Term Prognosis and Potential Complications *79*

CHAPTER 7
Effects on Family and Friends *105*

CHAPTER 8
Prevention *119*

CHAPTER 9
Issues and Controversies *129*

CHAPTER 10
Current Research and Future Directions *137*

Case Illustrations 145

Glossary 157

Directory of Resources 161

Bibliography 165

Index 173

Series Foreword

Disease is as old as humanity itself, and it has been the leading cause of death and disability throughout history. From the Black Death in the Middle Ages to smallpox outbreaks among Native Americans to the modern-day epidemics of diabetes and heart disease, humans have lived with—and died from—all manner of ailments, whether caused by infectious agents, environmental and lifestyle factors, or genetic abnormalities. The field of medicine has been driven forward by our desire to combat and prevent disease and to improve the lives of those living with debilitating disorders. And while we have made great strides forward, particularly in the last 100 years, it is doubtful that mankind will ever be completely free of the burden of disease.

Greenwood's Inside Diseases and Disorders series examines some of the key diseases and disorders, both physical and psychological, affecting the world today. Some (such as diabetes, cardiovascular disease, and ADHD) have been selected because of their prominence within modern America. Others (such as Ebola, celiac disease, and autism) have been chosen because they are often discussed in the media and, in some cases, are controversial or the subject of scientific or cultural debate.

Because this series covers so many different diseases and disorders, we have striven to create uniformity across all books. To maximize clarity and consistency, each book in the series follows the same format. Each begins with a collection of 10 frequently asked questions about the disease or disorder, followed by clear, concise answers. Chapter 1 provides a general introduction to the disease or disorder, including statistical information such as prevalence rates and demographic trends. The history of the disease or disorder, including how our understanding of it has evolved over time, is addressed in chapter 2. Chapter 3 examines causes and risk factors, whether genetic, microbial, or environmental, while chapter 4 discusses signs and symptoms. Chapter 5 covers the issues of diagnosis (and misdiagnosis), treatment, and management (whether with drugs, medical procedures, or lifestyle changes). How such treatment, or the lack thereof, affects a patient's long-term prognosis, as well as the risk of complications, are the subject of chapter 6. Chapter 7 explores the disease or disorder's effects on the friends and family of a patient—a dimension often overlooked in discussions of physical and psychological ailments. Chapter 8 discusses prevention strategies, while chapter 9 explores key issues or controversies, whether medical or sociocultural. Finally, chapter 10 profiles cutting-edge research and speculates on how things might change in the next few decades.

Each volume also features five fictional case studies to illustrate different aspects of the book's subject matter, highlighting key concepts and themes that have been explored throughout the text. The reader will also find a glossary of terms and a collection of print and electronic resources for additional information and further study.

As a final caveat, please be aware that the information presented in these books is no substitute for consultation with a licensed health care professional. These books do not claim to provide medical advice or guidance.

Acknowledgments

Although there is only one name on the cover of this book, many people have had a hand in helping it move from outline to completed manuscript. My thanks and appreciation are extended to my outstanding editor, Maxine Taylor, and the production staff at ABC-CLIO and Amnet for their patience and attention to detail. Thanks also to the Thursday Night Writers. Evelyn LaTorre, Jan Salinas, Joyce Cortez, and Loren and Claire Wright spent many evenings pointing out inconsistencies and confusing passages. This book is better because of them. Finally, without the support of my husband, Scott, and his patience in listening to me untangle thorny paragraphs, this book would not exist.

Introduction

Diabetes has reached near epidemic proportions. In 2017, 30.3 million Americans, or 9.4 percent of the population, were diabetic. The disorder is big business. One can hardly turn on the television without seeing advertisements for the latest glucose monitoring device or newest drugs to manage the disorder. In 2017, the United States spent 12 percent of all health care dollars—a whopping $727 billion—on diabetes care. These numbers are only expected to increase because 84.1 million American adults, or one-third of the population, have a condition called prediabetes. For many people, prediabetes will progress to full-blown type 2 diabetes.

The most common kind of diabetes, type 2 diabetes, is a stealthy disorder. Initially, it causes vague symptoms such as fatigue, increased thirst, and more frequent infections, all of which develop slowly and are often ignored. Even later symptoms such as blurred vision, cuts and bruises that are slow to heal, and numbness in the hands and feet tend to be blamed on aging. No wonder that, of the 30.3 million Americans with the disorder, almost one-quarter do not know they are affected, and many others find out they have the disorder only incidentally when they go to the doctor for a different complaint.

Worldwide, the situation is no better. The International Diabetes Foundation estimates that 425 million adults are diabetic. The greatest number of them are between 40 and 59 years old. Even more disturbing is that half the people with diabetes don't know they have the disorder and receive no treatment. The number of diabetics worldwide is projected to increase to 629 million by 2045, with the fastest rate of increase in low- and middle-income countries.

Diabetes can be confusing because it is not a single metabolic disorder. Only about 5 percent of diabetics have type 1 diabetes. Type 1 is an auto-immune disorder in which the body's immune system is triggered to attack and kill the cells that produce insulin. Insulin allows glucose, a simple sugar, to enter body cells where it powers all types of metabolic activities. No insulin means no cellular activity. Death results unless insulin is supplied from an outside source.

About 95 percent of diabetics have type 2 diabetes. Their bodies still make some insulin, but not enough, because their cells have become insulin resistant. Resistance makes it more difficult for glucose to enter cells. Left untreated, glucose builds up in the blood and causes complications throughout the body, such as increased risk of heart attack or stroke, nerve damage, kidney damage, and blindness.

A third type of diabetes, gestational diabetes, occurs in some women late in pregnancy and disappears once the baby is born. It is similar in effect to type 2 diabetes, although the causes are different, and complications can occur to both mother and baby.

This book examines the various types of diabetes, their causes, symptoms, and how and why they affect the mind and body. Of equal or more importance is information about steps to take that may prevent or delay diabetes and ways to manage the disorder. Diabetes has social effects in addition to physical ones. Effects on friends, family, and the workplace, along with economic costs of the disorder are discussed. Finally, research that offers hope for a cure, or if not a cure, better management of the disease is explored.

Essential Questions

1. WHAT ARE THE MAIN SYMPTOMS OF DIABETES?

The main symptoms of diabetes are increased thirst, increased urination, and excessive hunger. People with type 1 diabetes may also lose weight. These symptoms develop rapidly in type 1 diabetes and slowly in type 2 diabetes. Later symptoms of type 2 diabetes include fatigue; blurry vision; and cold, numb, or tingling hands and feet. Chapter 3 has more information about signs and symptoms. The diagnostic sign of diabetes is an elevated blood glucose (sugar) level.

2. WHAT IS THE DIFFERENCE BETWEEN TYPE 1 AND TYPE 2 DIABETES?

Only about 5 percent of diabetics have type 1 diabetes. Type 1 is an autoimmune disease in which the body's immune system destroys beta cells in the pancreas that produce insulin. Insulin is a hormone that allows the body to use glucose. Without insulin, glucose builds up in the blood. About 95 percent of diabetics have type 2 diabetes. These people make at least some insulin, but their cells have become insulin resistant, making it harder for glucose to get into the cells. Once again, glucose builds up in the blood. Chapter 1 provides more details about the different types of diabetes.

3. WHO IS MOST LIKELY TO GET DIABETES?

The risk of diabetes is not spread uniformly across the population. People who have a parent or sibling with type 1 diabetes are more likely to develop the disorder, although it can also arise spontaneously. Type 2 diabetes is strongly tied to obesity, an inactive lifestyle, and aging. There is also likely a genetic component, but it is difficult to determine because families share diets and lifestyles, as well as genetics. African Americans, Native Americans, Pacific Islanders, and people of Hispanic origin are at higher risk of developing type 2 diabetes. Chapter 3 discusses the risk factors for developing diabetes.

4. WHAT IS PREDIABETES?

Prediabetes is a condition in which blood glucose levels are above normal but not high enough to diagnose diabetes. Prediabetes is a warning sign that the individual is on the way to developing type 2 diabetes. The condition can sometimes be reversed through changes in diet and exercise. Chapter 1 describes the specifics of prediabetes, and chapter 8 discusses how it may be reversed.

5. WHAT IS GESTATIONAL DIABETES?

Gestational diabetes is abnormally high blood glucose that develops in some women late in pregnancy. It is caused by hormonal changes related to pregnancy and can be managed. Once the baby is born, glucose levels of the mother gradually return to normal. Some complications of gestational diabetes include giving birth to a very large baby and an increased risk of developing type 2 diabetes later in life. Chapters 1 and 6 have more information on gestational diabetes.

6. HOW IS DIABETES DIAGNOSED?

Diabetes is diagnosed by a simple blood test that measures blood glucose levels after an eight-hour fast. The exact numbers used to diagnose diabetes are in chapter 1, and a more extensive description of how the blood test is done appears in chapter 5.

7. HOW IS DIABETES TREATED?

Type 1 diabetes always requires treatment with injected insulin. There are many variations of insulin available, with different peaks of action and duration. Multiple classes of oral drugs are used to treat type 2 diabetes.

These drugs work in a variety of ways and have a range of side effects. Some stimulate the pancreas to make more insulin. Others slow the breakdown of insulin, and still others cause the liver to take up more glucose. The classes of drugs and their actions can be found in chapter 5.

8. WHAT ARE SOME OF THE COMPLICATIONS OF DIABETES?

Diabetes is a systemic disorder, meaning it can affect every part of the body. Common complications include an increased risk of stroke or heart attack, nerve damage in the legs and feet, vision loss, and slow wound healing. The disorder also can cause psychological complications, such as stress, depression, anxiety, and mood swings. Chapter 6 is devoted to complications.

9. CAN DIABETES BE CURED?

No. Many attempts have been made to cure diabetes, but, as of 2019, none have been successful. Chapter 10 details failed attempts to cure or prevent diabetes and looks at what may be in store for the future.

10. IS DIABETES RECOGNIZED AS A DISABILITY UNDER THE AMERICANS WITH DISABILITIES ACT?

Yes. Both type 1 and type 2 diabetes are recognized as disabilities under the Americans with Disabilities Act. The Act requires schools, workplaces, and other public spaces to make accommodations for people with diabetes. The federal act is supplemented and sometimes contradicted by state laws. Some accommodations and regulations are discussed in chapter 7.

1

What Is Diabetes?

Diabetes is formally called diabetes mellitus to distinguish it from diabetes insipidus, which is an unrelated disorder. Diabetes mellitus is not a single disease but refers to a group of related metabolic disorders that cannot be cured but can be effectively managed. All types of diabetes result in too much glucose (sugar) in the blood. This condition occurs from failure to produce any insulin, failure to produce adequate amounts of insulin, or failure of cells in the body to respond adequately to insulin. Insulin is the primary hormone that regulates glucose in the blood. Over time, hyperglycemia, an abnormally high level of blood glucose, also called high blood sugar, can damage many parts of the body, including the kidneys, heart, blood vessels, eyes, skin, feet, and nervous system. Left untreated, diabetes can cause fatal complications. Even though all types of diabetes result in high blood sugar levels, different types of diabetes have different causes and different treatments.

The two major types of diabetes are designated type 1 and type 2. Type 2 diabetes is far more common than type 1. Type 2 accounts for about 95 percent of people with the disorder. A condition called prediabetes often develops before type 2 diabetes and is a predictor for developing the disorder. Gestational diabetes is a form of diabetes that can develop during pregnancy, but, unlike the other types of diabetes, it is not a permanent condition. Researchers have also identified several rare forms of diabetes, including latent autoimmune diabetes in adults (LADA); monogenic

1

diabetes, which is caused by a rare gene mutation; chronic pancreatitis–associated diabetes; cystic fibrosis–related diabetes; and new-onset diabetes after organ transplantation. These forms of diabetes are uncommon.

BLOOD GLUCOSE REGULATION

Understanding how the body regulates the amount of glucose circulating in the blood is necessary to understanding diabetes and how it is treated. Glucose is a simple sugar made of carbon, hydrogen, and oxygen atoms. Almost all glucose in the body comes from carbohydrates in starchy foods, such as rice, pasta, bread, and potatoes, and sugar-heavy foods, such as cake, candy, fruit juice, and sugar- or fructose-sweetened sodas. When these foods are digested, they break down glucose and other molecules the body uses to build, repair, and maintain cells. Every cell in the body needs glucose for energy, but too much glucose in the blood causes diabetes.

For the body to function properly, it must maintain homeostasis. Homeostasis, derived from the ancient Greek words *homeo*, meaning "similar to," and *stasis*, meaning "standing still," is the condition of maintaining internal stability in the body. The way the body stays at a constant temperature even when the external temperature changes is an example of homeostasis.

In a healthy individual, a complex system of hormones and fluid regulation maintains homeostasis by keeping the level of blood glucose within the fairly narrow range of between 70 mg/dl (3.8 mmol/L) and 120 mg/dl (6.7 mmol/L), whether the individual has run a mile or eaten a feast.

When any of the mechanisms that tell the body how to handle glucose fail, glucose homeostasis is disrupted. If too much glucose builds up in the blood, a condition called hyperglycemia develops. With hyperglycemia, blood glucose concentrations stay above the normal level, and the individual develops diabetes. Without treatment, these high glucose levels damage many tissues and organs. If too little glucose is in the blood, a person develops hypoglycemia. Hypoglycemia can cause heart palpitations; confusion; seizures; loss of consciousness; and, if left untreated, death.

Table 1.1 compares blood glucose values for a healthy, nondiabetic person and the values used to diagnose prediabetes and diabetes. The international standard for measuring blood glucose levels is millimoles per liter, or mmol/L. The United States, Germany, and a few other countries measure blood sugar in milligrams per deciliter, or mg/dl. To convert mmol/L to mg/dl, multiply the mg/dl by 18. To convert mg/dl to mmol/L, divide the mg/dl by 18.

Table 1.1   Blood Glucose Values—Normal, Prediabetes, Diabetes

Time of Measurement	No Diabetes	Prediabetes	Diabetes
No food for at least 8 hours (fasting glucose test)	Less than 100 mg/dl (5.6 mmol/L)	100–125 mg/dl (5.6–7.0 mmol/L)	126 mg/dl (7.0 mmol/L) or higher
2 hours after drinking sugary liquid (oral glucose test)	Less than 140 mg/dl (7.8 mmol/L)	140–199 mg/dl (7.8 mmol/L–11.0 mmol/L)	200 mg/dl (11.1 mmol/L) or higher

THE PANCREAS

The pancreas is the master control organ for glucose regulation. It is a slightly flattened gland located behind the stomach on the upper left side of the body. In an adult, it is about 6 inches (15 cm) long and weighs about 3 ounces (85 g). The pancreas is both an exocrine gland and an endocrine gland.

Exocrine glands secrete fluids into ducts (tubules) that carry the fluid to another place in the body. Mammary glands that secrete milk are exocrine glands. Endocrine glands secrete hormones directly into the bloodstream. The testes, which secrete testosterone, are endocrine glands.

The pancreas is made up of both exocrine and endocrine cells. About 95 percent of the cells are exocrine cells. They secrete enzymes, water, and salts, collectively called pancreatic juice, into a duct that empties into the duodenum, which is the portion of the small intestine that is closest to the stomach. Almost 2 qt (2 L) of pancreatic juice are secreted every day. This fluid helps the body digest carbohydrates, fats, and proteins. Although important to health, the exocrine function of the pancreas and the digestive juices it produces have little to do with regulating blood glucose levels.

The endocrine cells of the pancreas regulate blood glucose levels. About three million endocrine cells are embedded in clumps within the exocrine tissue of the pancreas. These clumps are called the islets of Langerhans or simply pancreatic islets. They function independently of the exocrine gland cells and secrete the hormones that control glucose metabolism directly into a network of nearby blood vessels.

Pancreatic islets contain five different kinds of endocrine cells, each named by a Greek letter—alpha, beta, gamma, delta, and epsilon. Each type of cell produces different hormones that help keep the level of glucose in the blood within the narrow range needed to maintain health. About 20 percent of all islet cells are alpha cells, and 70 percent are beta cells. These two cell types have the strongest influence over blood glucose levels.

WHAT HAPPENS WHEN WE EAT?

When we eat, the digestive process breaks food down into small molecules that can be absorbed into the bloodstream from the small intestine. The breakdown of most food produces glucose, which is the energy source for all cells. Simple sugars, for example, sucrose (table sugar) and fructose (sugar in fruit), rapidly break down into glucose. Complex carbohydrates, which are in starchy foods, such as potatoes, rice, tortillas, and pasta, also break down into glucose and other molecules during the digestive process, but this takes a bit longer. The breakdown of fats and proteins creates some glucose along with other useful molecules, but the primary sources of glucose are simple sugars and complex carbohydrates.

When a food containing sugar or starch is eaten, the level of glucose in the blood begins to rise within 15–30 minutes and peaks in about 1.5 hours. The rise in blood sugar triggers beta cells in the pancreas to release a small protein hormone called insulin. The role of insulin is to reduce the amount of glucose in the blood. It does this in multiple ways.

• Insulin from the pancreas is secreted into the bloodstream and carried throughout the body. All cells have receptors for insulin embedded in their surface membranes. When insulin in the bloodstream meets a cell's insulin receptor, it binds to the receptor in a way that opens a channel for glucose to enter the cell. This allows the cell to renew its energy source and removes glucose from the blood. Brain cells are especially high users of glucose when a person is at rest. Skeletal muscle cells are high users of glucose when a person is physically active.

• At the same time, insulin acts rapidly on the liver, causing it to take in glucose and convert it into glycogen. Glycogen is made of a series of glucose molecules that are linked together. Creating glycogen allows glucose to be removed from the blood and be stored as reserve energy. When glucose levels are low, the liver can break down glycogen into glucose and release it into the bloodstream. Glycogen can make up as much as 10 percent of the weight of the liver in a person at rest.

• Insulin also acts on skeletal muscle cells to stimulate them to take up glucose and convert it into glycogen. Only about 2 percent of the weight of skeletal muscle is glycogen, but because the mass of skeletal muscle is much greater than that of the liver, most glycogen is stored in skeletal muscle. Insulin also acts on fat cells and stimulates them to take in excess glucose and convert it into fat.

• Insulin sends a message to the hypothalamus to suppress appetite, which, in turn, tells the individual to stop eating. The hypothalamus is a part of the brain that helps regulate the production of other hormones that affect basic body functions, such as body temperature, sex drive, sleep cycles, thirst, and appetite.

WHAT HAPPENS WHEN WE FAST?

Between meals or when we exercise, the body needs more glucose than is available in the blood. As blood glucose levels drop, alpha cells in the pancreatic islets secrete a hormone called glucagon. Glucagon has the opposite effect of insulin. It acts on receptors in the liver to cause chemical reactions that break down glycogen into glucose and release it into the bloodstream, where it circulates for use by other cells. Skeletal muscle cells can also break down glycogen into glucose, but they cannot release that glucose into the blood. Instead, they use this glucose as a source of energy for muscle cells during exercise.

OTHER PANCREATIC HORMONES

Insulin and glucagon are the yin and yang of blood sugar control. Insulin causes excess glucose to be removed from the blood. Glucagon causes glucose, stored as glycogen in the liver, to be released into the blood. Other pancreatic hormones, described below, have an important but much smaller effect on maintaining glucose homeostasis.

• Beta cells produce the hormone amylin in addition to insulin but in much smaller quantities. The ratio of insulin to amylin is about 100:1. This hormone was not discovered until 1987. Amylin slows glucagon secretion to keep blood sugar levels from getting too high. It also slows digestion, which reduces the speed at which glucose is absorbed into the bloodstream from the small intestine. When beta cells are damaged, both insulin and amylin production are severely reduced or absent. Without insulin, cells do not absorb glucose. At the same time, the lack of amylin takes the brake off glycogen conversion into glucose. As a result, the liver releases too much glucose into blood, where the glucose level is already too high.

- Delta cells secrete the hormone somatostatin. This hormone slows digestion and reduces the rate at which glucose is absorbed into the blood. Somatostatin is also secreted by the hypothalamus and the intestine.

- Epsilon cells secrete ghrelin. Ghrelin is a hormone that stimulates appetite and increases fat storage. Most ghrelin is made by the stomach, but small amounts are also made by epsilon cells in the pancreatic islets.

- Gamma cells, more commonly called PP cells, secrete a pancreatic polypeptide (a protein) that slows stomach emptying and reduces appetite. In animal studies, the absence of PP cells is associated with obesity. Obesity is a risk factor for type 2 diabetes.

TYPES OF DIABETES

It is important to understand how blood sugar levels are controlled because different types of diabetes develop from failures at different points in the glucose regulation system. Because failures occur at different points, the people more likely to develop each type of diabetes have different characteristics in terms of age, race, genetics, lifestyle factors, and effective treatments. Some of these differences are highlighted below and will be discussed in depth in future chapters.

Type 1 Diabetes

Type 1 diabetes was formerly called juvenile diabetes because it was most often diagnosed in young children. It was also called insulin-dependent diabetes because an external source of insulin is *absolutely required* for a person with type 1 diabetes to survive. Now that researchers better understand the varying causes of diabetes, the preferred name is type 1 diabetes.

Type 1 diabetes is an autoimmune disorder. Normally, immune system cells attack only viruses, bacteria that are foreign to the body, and abnormal human cells such as cancer cells. However, when a person has an autoimmune disorder, immune system cells misfire and attack and destroy normal, healthy body cells. In the case of type 1 diabetes, immune system cells attack and kill beta cells that produce insulin and amylin in the pancreas. Without insulin, glucose cannot enter cells, so it accumulates in the blood. Without amylin, the liver keeps converting glycogen into glucose to release into the bloodstream. The result is severe hyperglycemia that can only be brought under control by giving the individual insulin from an external source.

Type 1 diabetes occurs worldwide. Approximately 1.25 million Americans have type 1 diabetes, with about 40,000 new cases diagnosed each year. In the United Kingdom, approximately 400,000 people have the disorder, as do 300,000 Canadians. Type 1 diabetes is the most common metabolic disorder in children. Infrequently, the disorder can develop in adults, but most people are diagnosed before reaching adulthood.

Internationally, there is a big variation in the incidence of type 1 diabetes. For example, Finland has the highest incidence of type 1 diabetes at almost 65 persons per 100,000 population, while the rate in neighboring, Sweden, is only about 30 persons per 100,000 population. The incidence in the United States is about 24 per 100,000 population. China has a tiny incidence of 0.1 person per 100,000 population. Researchers cannot fully account for this wide variation. Genetics play a role, but so, apparently, do yet unidentified environmental factors. This is discussed more extensively in chapter 3.

Symptoms of type 1 diabetes suddenly become apparent only after about 80 percent of beta cells are destroyed. Symptoms include excessive thirst, excessive urination, extreme fatigue, blurred vision, and weight loss. Unlike people with type 2 diabetes, people with type 1 diabetes are rarely overweight. If unrecognized, symptoms can progress to a life-threatening condition called diabetic ketoacidosis (DKA). This occurs when not enough glucose is available to cells. Because glucose cannot enter cells, the body begins to break down fat to use for energy. As fat is broken down, it produces molecules called ketones. Ketones make blood more acidic, which throws off the biochemical balance of the body. DKA is a medical emergency. Untreated, it can result in nausea, vomiting, acetone-smelling breath, weakness, coma, and death.

Diabetes is easy to diagnose through simple blood tests, but in children the signs of type 1 diabetes are often missed or are suspected of having other origins. Once type 1 diabetes is diagnosed, the only effective treatment is to provide insulin from an external source (originally from pig or calf pancreas, and now laboratory-produced) multiple times each day. The dose must be calculated based on the diet and activity level of the individual and is injected directly into the body, because insulin given by mouth will be destroyed by stomach acids.

Type 2 Diabetes

Type 2 diabetes used to be called adult-onset diabetes because most people who developed type 2 diabetes were over the age of 45. However, children and young adults are increasingly developing type 2 diabetes. Type 2 diabetes also used to be called non-insulin-dependent diabetes because insulin from an external source was not absolutely required for survival. Today many people with long-standing type 2 diabetes do require insulin in addition to lifestyle changes and other medications to control their blood sugar levels, so the name non-insulin-dependent diabetes is no longer used.

In 2018, about 30.3 million Americans, or 9.4 percent of the population, had diabetes. This compares to 1 percent of the population in 1958. Approximately 95 percent have type 2 diabetes, but only about 23.1 million know that they have the disorder. Another 7.2 million have blood glucose levels that are high enough to be diagnosed with diabetes, but they have not been tested, which means they are not receiving any treatment.

Worldwide, about 425 million people, or one out of every eleven adults, are estimated to have type 2 diabetes. Certain ethnic and cultural groups are more likely to develop the disorder. In the United States, the prevalence of type 2 diabetes is 77 percent higher in Latinos, 66 percent higher in African Americans, and 20 percent higher in Asian Americans than in non-Latino whites. Pacific Islanders, Native Americans, and Native Hawaiians also have very high rates of type 2 diabetes.

Genetic inheritance appears to play a bigger role in the development of type 2 diabetes than in type 1 diabetes. If one parent has type 2 diabetes, there is a 40 percent chance that their child will develop the disorder. If both parents have type 2 diabetes, the risk rises to 70 percent, and if one identical twin has the disorder, there is also a 70 percent chance that the other twin will also have type 2 diabetes. Genetic inheritance, however, is only one risk factor for developing type 2 diabetes. Other major risk factors include being overweight or obese, getting little physical exercise, and being over the age of 45 years. These are discussed more extensively in chapter 3.

The cause of type 2 diabetes differs from type 1. In type 2 diabetes, chemical changes in the body make it harder for glucose to enter cells, including liver, fat, and muscle cells where excess glucose is stored for future use. In other words, insulin no longer easily triggers the opening of a gateway for glucose to enter cells. This insensitivity to insulin is called insulin resistance. Beta cells remain intact, but they do not make enough insulin to allow adequate glucose uptake by cells. Type 2 diabetes is a progressive disorder. Over time, the amount of insulin beta cells make decreases, while the amount of glucagon produced by alpha cells may increase, causing worsening of hyperglycemia.

The symptoms of type 2 diabetes are similar to those of type 1—excessive thirst, excessive urination, extreme fatigue, blurred vision—but often with little or no weight loss. The main difference is that these symptoms develop gradually and are often unrecognized, which is why so many people with type 2 diabetes remain undiagnosed and untreated.

Blood glucose levels in people with type 2 diabetes can often be controlled or kept from worsening by changes in diet, increased exercise, and non-insulin medication. Treatment and management of diabetes are discussed in chapter 5.

Prediabetes

Prediabetes, sometimes called impaired glucose tolerance or intermediate hyperglycemia, is not diabetes, but it is an important set of warning signs that a person is on the road to developing type 2 diabetes within a few years. Prediabetes is diagnosed when blood glucose levels are not low enough to determine that the individual does not have diabetes, but they are also not high enough to diagnose and treat the person for type 2 diabetes (see Table 1.1). Along with higher-than-normal blood glucose, people with prediabetes often have hypertension (high blood pressure), high levels of low-density lipoprotein (LDL) or "bad" cholesterol, a high level of triglycerides (fats in the blood), and are overweight or obese.

The U.S. Centers for Disease Control and Prevention (CDC) estimated that in 2017, one of every three Americans—about 84.1 million people—had prediabetes. Of these, about 23 million were age 65 or older. The bad news is that about 70 percent of people with prediabetes will eventually develop type 2 diabetes. The good news is that this is not inevitable. With lifestyle changes, the risk of a person with prediabetes progressing to diabetes can be reduced by between 40 and 70 percent. Even for those people who do eventually develop type 2 diabetes, the progression of the disorder can be delayed. The most important lifestyle changes for reversing prediabetes are losing weight; eating healthy, well-balanced meals, and getting regular moderate exercise.

Gestational Diabetes

Gestational diabetes is diabetes that develops only when a woman becomes pregnant. It is not the same as having diabetes before becoming pregnant. Gestational diabetes occurs in between 2 and 10 percent of pregnancies. Like type 2 diabetes, the occurrence of gestational diabetes is strongly related to ethnicity and culture. Gestational diabetes occurs in only about 2 percent of pregnancies of women of European ancestry. It is four to five times higher in African American, Asian, and Latina women. In some Native American populations, the rate is as high as 15 percent.

During pregnancy, hormones produced by the placenta make cells in the body less sensitive to insulin. This is a normal result of pregnancy, and it allows more glucose to circulate to the fetus, where it is used for growth. As pregnancy progresses and the fetus grows, the placenta produces more and more anti-insulin hormones. In a woman who develops gestational diabetes, the placental hormones overwhelm the amount of insulin she can make, and her cells become resistant to glucose. The level of glucose in her blood rises and stays high. She soon develops hyperglycemia and symptoms of diabetes. There is no known way to prevent this.

Women who are obese, have a family history of type 2 diabetes, have been diagnosed with prediabetes, or have had gestational diabetes with a previous pregnancy, all of which are risk factors for developing the disorder, are given blood glucose tests early in pregnancy. All other women are screened at between 24 and 28 weeks of pregnancy because this is the time when gestational diabetes usually develops in low-risk women.

Gestational hyperglycemia also has consequences for the fetus, including excessive weight gain while in the uterus. Women with gestational diabetes often give birth to babies weighing 9 pounds (4.1 kg) or more. Additional short- and long-term complications for mother and child are discussed in chapter 6.

Gestational diabetes is treated with a carefully planned diet; appropriate exercise; and, if necessary, medication and insulin. Fortunately, gestational diabetes is not permanent. Once the baby is born, the mother's blood glucose level usually drops to near normal after a few weeks, especially if she is breast-feeding. However, a woman who has had gestational diabetes is at much higher risk of developing type 2 diabetes relatively early in life.

THE COST OF DIABETES

Diabetes is big business. You can hardly turn on the television without seeing an advertisement for diabetes testing supplies or insulin, along with drugs to treat type 2 diabetes or slow its progression. A study by the American Diabetes Association (ADA) found that in 2017, diabetes cost Americans $237 billion in direct medical costs. Approximately one of every seven dollars spent on health care went to treating diabetes or its complications. The average cost of insulin alone was $450 per month. In addition to direct health care costs, an estimated $90 billion was lost in reduced productivity, an increase of 26 percent in just five years.

Worldwide, the cost of diabetes was estimated in 2017 to be $825 billion per year, and the costs are rising as the number of people with diabetes increases. The ADA also found that in 2017, people diagnosed with diabetes spent an average of $16,750 on medical expenses, of which $9,600 was directly attributed to diabetes. This was 2.3 times more than the medical expenditures of people without diabetes. Comparisons of the cost of some types of insulin and insulin delivery systems for people without insurance as of late 2019 can be found at https://www.goodrx.com/blog/how-much-does-insulin-cost-compare-brands/.

Diabetes also has quality-of-life costs. These include blindness, kidney failure, increased susceptibility to heart attack and stroke, nerve damage, poor wound healing, amputation, and disabilities that prevent individuals from working or enjoying life. In 2018, diabetes was the seventh-leading cause of death in the United States, although this ranking is thought to seriously underrepresent the role of diabetes in contributing to other causes of death. Diabetes also shortens life spans. The ADA also estimated that the disorder caused 277,000 premature deaths in the United States in 2017. In the United Kingdom, the National Health Service estimated that each week 500 people with diabetes die prematurely.

2

The History of Diabetes

Some signs of the disorder we now call diabetes mellitus—excessive thirst, production of copious sweet-smelling urine, and severe weight loss—have been recognized for centuries, and for centuries, these signs telegraphed a death sentence. Frustrated physicians tried any number of ways to treat or cure the disorder. Not until the discovery of insulin was there hope for survival after a diagnosis of diabetes. Even though insulin and other medications can effectively control the symptoms of diabetes today, there remains no cure for the disorder.

DIABETES IN ANCIENT TIMES

The oldest description of diabetes was unearthed from an Egyptian tomb in the mid-1800s. The manuscript, known as the Ebers Papyrus, was written in about 1550 BCE. It is the most extensive collection of medical knowledge about diseases and treatments that we have from that time period. In it, the writer describes the frequent and excessive urination that is a sign of diabetes and recommends treatment with a mixture of "Water from a Bird Pond, Elderberry, Fibres of the asit plant, Fresh Milk, Beer-Swill, Flower of Cucumber, and Green Dates" (Sanders 2002, 56).

Around the same time that the Ebers Papyrus was written, physicians in India noticed that ants were attracted to the urine of people who had excessive thirst and bad breath and who produced an extreme volume of urine. They did not understand why ants liked this urine, but today we know it is because the urine of untreated diabetics contains a high concentration of sugar, a condition called glycosuria. Indian physicians called urine that attracted ants "madhumeha" which translates as "honey urine." Checking whether ants were attracted to urine became the first diagnostic test for diabetes, although diagnosis did not lead to any effective treatment. People with the disorder still drank gallons of water, urinated almost constantly, lost large amounts of weight (a second-century Greek physician described the phenomenon as flesh melting into urine), lapsed into a coma, and died.

Although symptoms of diabetes were recognized throughout the ancient world, the first person to actually give the name "diabetes" to the disorder was an Egyptian physician named Apollonius of Memphis, who lived around 230 CE. He combined two Greek words—*dia*, meaning "through" and *betes*, meaning "to go" to describe the excessive flow of urine out of the body. He and other physicians of that time believed that diabetes was a disease of the kidneys.

UNDERSTANDING OF DIABETES STALLS

For the next 1,300 years, almost no progress was made in understanding diabetes. Treatments remained just as odd and ineffective as they were in ancient Egypt. Finally, in the sixteenth century, the Swiss physician Paracelsus (1493–1541) found that when he evaporated urine from people with diabetes, a residue of whitish crystals remained. He believed these were salts from the kidney. He thought the "salts" caused excessive thirst and water intake. The residue was finally correctly identified in 1776 by British physiologist Matthew Dobson (ca. 1732–1784) who determined that it was sugar. Dobson also noticed the sweet taste of blood serum in people with diabetes. This caused him to suggest that the symptoms he observed were systemic and not limited to the kidneys.

At about the same time that Dobson identified sugar in the urine of diabetics, Scottish physician William Cullen (1710–1790) added the word "mellitus," from the Latin word for "honey" to the description of diabetes to distinguish the disorder from diabetes insipidus. Diabetes insipidus also causes the production of large quantities of urine, but the urine does not contain sugar. This disorder results from failure of the pituitary gland to secrete the antidiuretic hormone vasopressin or failure of the body to respond to that hormone. It is not related to diabetes mellitus.

EXPERIMENTATION AND OBSERVATION

The 1800s in Europe were a time of intense interest in the biochemistry and physiology of body functions. In 1815, French scientist Michel-Eugène Chevreul (1786–1889) identified the type of sugar in the urine of diabetics as the simple sugar glucose. German chemist Hermann von Fehling (1812–1885) then developed a test to measure glucose in urine. This test gave physicians a way to definitively diagnose diabetes. In addition, as the century progressed, physicians became more aware of the various complications diabetes causes in multiple parts of the body. These complications are discussed in chapter 6.

Some of the experiments that scientists performed led almost accidentally to an increased knowledge about the cause of diabetes. Until 1848, the role of the pancreas was unknown. While studying the digestive tract, French physiologist Claude Bernard (1813–1878) discovered that the pancreas produced digestive enzymes that flowed through a duct into the small intestine. Using dogs to experiment, he tied off the pancreatic duct to stop the movement of these enzymes. This created digestive problems, but the dogs did not develop diabetes or die. Bernard also isolated glycogen in the liver and realized it could be broken down and released into the blood as glucose. This observation became important in understanding how the amount of sugar in the blood is regulated.

A few years later, when Paul Langerhans (1847–1888) studied the pancreas for his doctoral dissertation, he noticed that it contained clumps of different-appearing cells that did not drain into the pancreatic duct. These clumps of cells are now called the islets of Langerhans in his honor. Langerhans reported the odd cell clumps, but he had no idea of their function and did not pursue this question.

As late as 1889, it still was unclear that the pancreas had anything to do with diabetes. However, in that year, Oskar Minkowski (1858–1931) and Joseph von Mering (1849–1908), working at Strasbourg University, removed the entire pancreas from a dog. The dog developed all the symptoms of diabetes and died. They repeated the experiment on more dogs with the same result. They then removed the pancreas but implanted a small piece of it under each dog's skin where it was not connected to the pancreatic duct. These dogs remained relatively healthy until the implanted piece of pancreas was removed, after which they developed diabetes symptoms and died. Minkowski and von Mering's experiments showed that something in the pancreas was necessary for normal glucose regulation. Five years later, French pathologist Gustave-Édouard Laguesse (1861–1927) suggested that the critical substance came from the odd clumps of cells discovered by Paul Langerhans.

THE ALLEN DIET

In the United States, research interest turned to the role of diet in health. Physician Frederick Allen (1876–1964) initially began studying the effects of sugar consumption but soon shifted to doing diabetes experiments on dogs at Harvard University. Over the course of 10 years of experimentation, he found that if he removed 20 percent of the pancreas, experimental dogs did not become diabetic. If he removed 80–90 percent of the pancreas, some dogs developed symptoms of diabetes while others did not. The severity of the symptoms depended on the dogs' diet. Dogs fed a low-carbohydrate diet remained relatively healthy. Dogs fed a high-carbohydrate diet developed diabetes. These findings suggested to Allen that humans with diabetes could be helped with a low-carbohydrate diet.

When Allen moved to Rockefeller Institute Hospital in New York in 1914, he treated people with severe diabetes by having them fast for several days and then eat a very low-carbohydrate/low-calorie diet that is usually referred to as a starvation diet. This diet, he believed, would keep blood glucose levels low and improve diabetes symptoms. Some patients soon died, while others lived longer than expected on the very low-calorie diet. Allen noted that the death rate in patients under the age of 30 was much higher than in those aged 40 and older, although he did not know what this meant. Based on what we know today, this likely reflected whether the patient had type 1 or type 2 diabetes; however, the existence of two types of diabetes was not formally suggested until 1936.

Allen's starvation diet was highly controversial, and its use divided the diabetes clinic staff at the hospital into pro-Allen and anti-Allen camps. In the end, Allen, to his intense frustration, was removed from a position of authority in the diabetes clinic. His association with Rockefeller Institute ended when he was inducted into the army and sent to treat patients at a diabetes facility in Lakewood, New Jersey.

Returning to civilian life in 1919, Allen, now a recognized diabetes expert, established a private practice in New York to treat diabetic children with his starvation diet. Unlike the many swindlers who peddled diabetes "cures," Allen never claimed that he could cure diabetes, only that his diet would extend life long enough for a cure to be found.

The diet was rigorous. Patients were often limited to 500 calories per day or less. (The recommended caloric intake for an active 10-year-old boy today is 2,200 calories.) Every morsel of food had to be weighed and measured. Blood glucose levels were checked several times every day so that the calorie allowance could be adjusted. Some patients died of starvation. Many others simply could not stand the pain of starvation, abandoned the diet, and died when their blood glucose rose.

One of Allen's patients at this time was Elizabeth Hughes (1907–1981). Elizabeth's father was the politically prominent Charles Evans Hughes (1862–1948), former governor of New York and later a Supreme Court justice. In 1916, Hughes resigned from the Supreme Court to run for president against Woodrow Wilson, a race he narrowly lost. When Elizabeth developed diabetes symptoms at the age of 11, her parents consulted Allen. After agonizing over the decision, they agreed to put her on the Allen diet and had a nurse specially trained to prepare her food, monitor her blood glucose, and serve as her companion. When Elizabeth began the diet, she weighed 75 pounds (34 kg). During her time on the diet, she grew to be five feet (152 cm) tall, while her weight dropped to a skeletal 48 pounds (21 kg).

Frederick Allen was dedicated to treating diabetic children and had the vision of establishing a residential institution where these children could be treated, regardless of their ability to pay. He enlisted Elizabeth's father to create a committee to raise funds for the project. Charles Hughes then used his social and political connections to solicit other wealthy men to support the project. In 1920, Allen used the money Hughes raised to purchase an estate in Morristown, New Jersey, and established the Physiatric Institute. Here he devoted himself to extending the lives of diabetic children, always hoping that a cure would become available before they died of the disorder or from the effects of starvation. A cure never materialized, but a lifesaving breakthrough was not far away.

THE FARM BOY

While Frederick Allen was busy prolonging life at the Physiatric Institute, Frederick Banting (1891–1941), a young Canadian doctor, was struggling with a return to civilian life after World War I ended. Banting had grown up on a farm in Alliston, Ontario. The youngest of five children, he was expected to do as his brothers had done and drop out of school after the eighth grade to farm full time. Instead, to the dismay of his family, he finished high school and went to the University of Toronto, where he earned a medical degree in 1916. The decision to choose medicine over farm life was something his family could not understand, and ,for years while he did research and made very little money, they considered him a failure.

Immediately after receiving his medical degree, Banting enlisted in the Canadian Army Medical Corps. He was sent to France, where he served as a surgeon near the front lines, amputating limbs and stabilizing wounded soldiers so that they could be evacuated to safer locations. During his service, he was wounded and received the Military Cross for heroism under fire.

Returning to Canada after the war, Banting studied for a year at the University of Toronto to qualify as an orthopedic surgeon. He then borrowed money from his family to buy a house and open a medical practice in London, Ontario. Banting was an introvert and often felt awkward and inferior around others who had grown up in socially prominent, well-educated families. With his lack of social skills, his new practice attracted very few patients, his debts piled up, and the fiancée who had promised to wait for him while he was at war had second thoughts about marriage. Finally, financial pressures forced Banting to take a part-time position as a lecturer at the University of Western Ontario at a very low salary. This was not the life he had envisioned when he went to medical school.

BANTING'S LIFE-CHANGING IDEA

On the night of October 31, 1920, Banting happened to read a journal article by American pathologist Moses Barron (1884–1974), in which Barron described an unusual situation he had encountered during an autopsy. In the article, he described how calcified material had blocked the pancreatic duct. As a result of the blockage, all the cells that produced digestive enzymes had died, leaving mainly islet cells. Banting was not particularly interested in the pancreas, and the article put him to sleep, but when he awoke from his nap, he had an idea. In his notebook he wrote in his usual poor spelling,

> Diabetus [sic] Ligate pancreatic ducts of dog. Keep dogs alive till acini [the cells producing digestive enzymes] degenerate leave Islets. Try to isolate the internal secretions of these to relieve glycosurea [sic]. (Bliss 2007, 50)

After this insight, Banting became obsessed with the idea. He was convinced that it would produce a medical breakthrough that would cure hyperglycemia and prove to his family that he was not a failure.

THE SCOTSMAN

While Banting was attending medical school, serving in the army, and struggling to develop a medical practice, John James Rickard Macleod (1876–1935) had acquired a reputation as an outstanding physiologist and biochemist. After completing his medical education in Scotland, Macleod won a research scholarship and moved to the United States, where he became a professor of physiology at Western Reserve University (now Case Western University) in Cleveland, Ohio. His area of research was carbohydrate metabolism, and he wrote a book on diabetes.

Despite working in the United States, Macleod remained intensely loyal to Great Britain. He saw the effects of World War I (1914–1918) on friends and family still living there and was angered that, in his view, the United States was dragging its feet in support of the war effort. (The United States did not enter the war until April 1917). Acting on his patriotic anger, Macleod moved to Canada, which, as part of the British Empire, had sent troops to fight in Europe as soon as the war began. Macleod soon became an influential professor of physiology and assistant to the dean of the medical school at the University of Toronto.

When Frederick Banting proposed his idea for isolating an active ingredient in islet cells to a friend at Western Ontario University, the friend referred him to J. J. R. Macleod in Toronto. Banting and Macleod came from completely different social backgrounds and had different perspectives on the purpose of medical research. Macleod wanted to advance scientific knowledge. Banting wanted to develop clinical applications that would save lives. Putting them together was like mixing oil and water.

FINDING A SPONSOR

Frederick Banting met J. J. R. Macleod in November 1920, one week after having his brainstorm about extracting material from islet cells to treat diabetes. Banting wanted Macleod and the University of Toronto to give him funding and laboratory space to test his idea. Macleod knew little about Banting except that he was an alumnus of the university's medical school and had served as a surgeon during the war, but he agreed to meet with him.

The meeting got off to a poor start. Macleod was 15 years older than Banting, expensively dressed, confident of his position at the university, and an expert in carbohydrate metabolism. Banting was full of enthusiasm for his idea but poorly dressed, nervous, self-conscious, and inarticulate. Macleod was not impressed. For one thing, Macleod was familiar with the work of Minkowski, von Mering, and others who had tried and failed to do what Banting proposed. He sent Banting away, telling him to do a literature search and write a research proposal if he wanted his idea to be considered by the university.

Banting was offended that Macleod did not see the brilliance of his idea. He returned home in a huff, but by March his annoyance had lessened, and his debts increased, so he wrote the required letter. In response, Macleod, who planned to spend the summer in Scotland, offered Banting lab space, a student assistant, and a few dogs to experiment on for two months during the summer. Neither Banting nor his student assistant would receive a salary or living expenses.

A FRUSTRATING BEGINNING

The space Macleod provided was not the gleaming laboratory Banting had envisioned. The room was hot and dirty. The wooden operating table could not be sterilized, and the floor could not be scrubbed, because water leaked through it into the room below. Cleanliness was essential to preventing infection in this era before antibiotics, especially in areas where surgery was performed.

Macleod introduced Banting to two medical students, Charles Best (1899–1978) and Clark Noble (1900–1978), who were to be his assistants. Banting needed only one assistant, so the students decided that each would work for one month. The men tossed a coin and determined that Best would assist first. As it turned out, Best stayed for the entire summer and beyond.

Macleod gave Banting 12 dogs for experimentation. Two dogs were needed for each experiment. A donor dog would have its pancreatic duct tied off so that the enzyme-producing cells would die. The reason for this was the mistaken idea that enzymes in the digestive part of the pancreas would inactivate the substance in the islet cells. After a few weeks, the remaining islet-rich tissue would be removed. Best, whose background was in biochemistry, would mash up and chemically treat the islet tissue to extract a substance that Banting named isletin. This was the magic substance he expected would control hyperglycemia.

To test the extract, a second dog, the recipient dog, would have its pancreas completely removed so that it became diabetic. This dog would then be injected with the islet cell extract, and its blood glucose and urine glucose measured. If glucose levels dropped, this would show that something in the islet cells affected how the body used glucose.

The project got off to a rough start. Macleod demonstrated the technique of tying off the pancreatic duct for Banting and then left for Scotland. The surgery was tricky. Banting, whose surgical experience was with humans, flubbed the first two canine operations. A third dog died of infection. Already Banting was down to nine dogs with two months of research time remaining. Later, whenever Banting and Best ran out of dogs, they scoured Toronto at night to collect strays for their experiments.

Failure followed failure. In some donor dogs, the pancreatic duct was not tied off tightly enough. The pancreas did not atrophy, so the surgery had to be repeated. Dogs died not just from intentionally induced diabetes but from overdoses of anesthesia, infection, and surgical error. In addition, the extract Best produced worked inconsistently. Sometimes it lowered blood glucose the first time it was injected but was ineffective when the injection was repeated. After weeks of work, there were no reliable results to report. Banting was discouraged but determined.

A HINT OF SUCCESS

Toward the end of the summer, there was a glimmer of success. The lab kept a collie, whose pancreas had been removed, alive for 19 days using the extract from donor dogs' pancreases. The collie remained healthy as long as it was given injections of extract, but when the extract ran out, the collie became diabetic and died. Banting sent news of the collie's survival time to Macleod in Scotland along with a demand for things he required to continue his work into the autumn. These included a salary, a person to care for the dogs, a room to work in, and repair of the laboratory floor.

Macleod's response was to remind Banting that one success was not adequate proof of his theory. He completely ignored the demand list. Banting took this to mean that Mcleod did not have faith in the work the lab was doing. Even so, Banting had so much confidence in his idea (and had become so poor) that he returned to London, Ontario, sold his heavily mortgaged house, furniture, and medical equipment in a single day, and relocated permanently to Toronto.

When Macleod returned from Scotland, Banting threatened go to another institution unless his situation improved. Macleod then met some of Banting's demands, including a dog caretaker and a workroom. He refused to fix the laboratory floor but did find a new space where Banting could operate. He did not offer Banting a salary but paid him only $150 ($2,130 in 2018 Canadian dollars) for his summer's work, while paying Best, the assistant, $170 ($2,410 in 2018 CAD). On his own initiative, Banting found a part-time job as an assistant in the pharmacology department. From this point forward, the relationship between Banting and Macleod went downhill.

CONFLICTS AND MISUNDERSTANDINGS

Work continued in the lab, with some failures but also more successes. In November 1921, Macleod suggested that Banting present his preliminary research findings to a group of students who belonged to the university's Physiological Journal Club. At this meeting, Macleod was supposed to introduce Banting but instead of a simple introduction, Macleod went on to describe all the work Banting had intended to talk about. In describing the research, Macleod used the terms "we" and "our," as if he had been in the lab all summer with Banting and Best rather than vacationing in Scotland. Banting, never a good public speaker, was left tongue-tied and embarrassed with nothing further to say. Although Banting did not confront Macleod about upstaging him, he was furious that the man appeared to take credit for work he and Best had done.

Soon after this incident, Banting had a breakthrough that accelerated his research. It had been assumed that the enzyme-producing part of the pancreas had to be destroyed so as not to harm the glycemic control substance in the islet cells. Tying off the pancreatic duct and waiting four to seven weeks for the enzyme-producing tissue to die limited how fast experimentation could proceed. Banting had read that a French pathologist discovered islet cells were especially abundant in fetal animals. Perhaps, Banting thought, since the digestive tract does not begin to function until after birth, fetal pancreases might not contain destructive enzymes. If this were true, whole fresh fetal pancreas could be ground up, and the isletin extracted.

From growing up on a farm, Banting knew that farmers often bred their cows before slaughter because pregnancy increased their appetite and made them gain weight. He visited a slaughterhouse and acquired some fresh fetal pancreases. The fresh extract worked even better than the extract from atrophied pancreases. (Later it would be shown that adult fresh pancreases could also be used. The precursors of the destructive enzymes were present in fresh pancreases but were not activated until they entered the digestive system.) Suddenly, the team had an abundant source of pancreases and no longer had to depend on donor dogs.

ATTEMPTS TO EXPAND

James Bertram Collip (1892–1965), a brilliant biochemist from the University of Alberta, appeared on the scene in the summer of 1921. Collip's research was on glands of internal secretion, such as the pancreas. He had been awarded a prestigious Rockefeller Fellowship that allowed him to study for a year at institutions of his choice. His intention was to work at the University of Toronto for a few months, and then move on to laboratories in New York and London. Instead, he became interested in Banting and Best's work and stayed in Toronto.

Collip wanted to work with Banting and Best, but despite multiple requests from both Collip and Banting, when Macleod returned from Scotland, he refused to include Collip, saying that it was too soon to expand the team. Banting took Macleod's refusal as yet another sign that he had no faith in the lab's research. Eventually, after Banting began to get positive results, Macleod allowed Collip to join the team with the task of improving Best's process for purifying and concentrating isletin.

UPSTAGED AGAIN

By December 1921, Banting and Best finally had enough material to write a research paper. The paper was to be published by a journal in

February, but before then, Banting and Best were to present their findings at the American Physiological Society conference at Yale University. The conference attracted some of the most famous diabetes researchers in the United States and Canada. Macleod was president of the society. Banting and Best were not even members. Consequently, to draw attention to the research, Macleod's name was included as an author on the presentation.

Banting was a poor public speaker under the best of circumstances, and the crowd of experts at the conference made him nervous. He spoke haltingly, often lowering his voice and mumbling. In the question period following his talk, Banting fell apart. He later admitted, "I became almost paralyzed. I could not remember nor could I think" (Bliss 2007, 104). At that point, Macleod took over answering the questions, once again using "we" and "our" to refer to experiments he had not directly participated in. Back in Toronto, when Banting recovered from his humiliation, he was furious. He believed that Macleod was stealing credit for his and Best's work.

THE FIRST PATIENT

Banting and Best continued to try to improve the purity of the pancreatic extract, while Collip, working in a different building with Macleod, tried to do the same. A feeling of competition rather than collaboration developed. Because Banting was primarily interested in the clinical application of his research, he convinced Dr. Walter Campbell, director of the diabetes clinic at Toronto General Hospital, to try his extract on a patient. Campbell chose 14-year-old Leonard Thompson as the trial patient.

Thompson was on the Allen diet, weighed 65 pounds (29.5 kg), and was failing fast. On January 11, 1922, he received an injection of Banting and Best's extract, inaccurately recorded in the patient's records as "Macleod's Serum." However, Campbell refused to allow Banting to give the shot, even though he was the only practicing physician on the research team. Instead, he insisted that a house physician give the shot, with the added insult that the diabetes clinic refused to give Banting any urine or blood samples for testing, insisting that glucose levels could only be tested by the hospital laboratory.

When the results came back, they showed a minimal decrease in the amount of sugar in Thompson's blood and urine. The boy also developed a painful sore at the injection site, probably in reaction to impurities in the extract. The clinic director ruled that results were not significant enough to justify another shot. Banting was both angry and demoralized, and things were about to get worse.

A PHYSICAL CONFRONTATION

A few days later, Collip strolled into Banting and Best's lab and announced that he had found a way to completely purify the pancreatic extract. When Banting asked how he had done it, Collip replied that he and Macleod had decided not to tell Banting and Best. Then he announced that he was going to leave the research group and take out a patent on the process in his own name. That was too much for Banting who, with Best, had developed the foundation for the extraction process that Collip then improved. Banting sprang across the room and physically attacked Collip. Best had to separate the men before one of them was seriously hurt.

Two positive things developed out of this confrontation. First, it became clear that the extract had commercial possibilities. As a result, an agreement was drafted and signed by Banting, Best, Collip, and Macleod stating that they would not take any steps to patent or commercially develop the extract; commercial development was to be done by the University of Toronto. Second, when Leonard Thompson was treated with Collip's newly purified extract, his blood and urine glucose levels dropped significantly. With continued injections, he put on weight and regained strength. With regular insulin shots, Thompson lived another 13 years and died of pneumonia.

For the next four months, experiments continued using Collip's extract on dogs, rabbits, and unofficially on a few humans. (Banting and Best were said to have injected each other to see what would happen). Meanwhile, Banting suffered an apparent breakdown. His extract had not performed well, his on-again-off-again engagement appeared to be off permanently, and he felt shut out of decisions that Macleod and Collip were making in the lab. By his own admission, Banting did little work and spent most of March drunk. Years later he wrote, "Best and I became technicians under Macleod . . . Neither plans for experiments nor results were discussed with us" (Bliss 2007, 121). Finally, a confrontation with Best, who threatened to leave the team if Banting did not return, prodded him to stop drinking and return to work.

THE WORLD IS INTRODUCED TO INSULIN

The University of Toronto had established the Connaught Anti-Toxin Laboratory in 1914 to make anti-diphtheria toxin and vaccines. In early 1922, it was decided that this laboratory would make the pancreatic extract, still called isletin, under Collip's direction. Then the almost unimaginable happened.

Collip had not written down the purification process and lost the ability to purify and concentrate the extract. He worked furiously to try to reproduce what he had done in January and February, with little success. Banting blamed Collip for refusing to share his extraction technique with the research team. This led to another physically violent public incident between Banting and Collip. At this point, the two men could not safely be in the same room.

Collip finally regained his extraction mojo, and, by spring the team had enough experimental data for a major presentation. At this time, Macleod requested that the name of the extract, called isletin by Banting, be changed to insulin. On April 22, 1922, a patent on insulin was issued in the names of Best and Collip to prevent others from commercially exploiting their work. They were chosen because they were not medical doctors; Best was a student and Collip had a PhD. In the 1920s, the medical community considered it improper for doctors to work with pharmaceutical companies on for-profit drugs. Best and Collip immediately signed the patent over to the University of Toronto for one dollar.

On May 3, 1922, Macleod presented the team's research results at the Association of American Physicians conference in Washington, D.C. Banting and Best did not attend the conference. It was immediately clear to all present that the results were what one attendee called "epoch-making." It had taken only 50 weeks from Banting and Best's first experiments in the dirty, inadequate laboratory that Macleod had assigned them to develop, with the help of an enlarged team, a pancreatic extract that could save the lives of people with diabetes.

SCALING UP PRODUCTION

Newspapers enthusiastically reported on the insulin breakthrough, sometimes incorrectly calling it a "cure" for diabetes. Dozens of diabetics went to Toronto, hoping that would increase their chances of receiving the drug. Thousands of others or their doctors wrote, begging for insulin. Getting access to the drug could quite literally mean the difference between life and death. Connaught Laboratory could not keep up with demand, and most people requesting the drug had to be turned down.

At this point, George Clowes (1877–1958), representing the pharmaceutical company Eli Lilly, approached the board of governors of the University of Toronto, which now controlled the insulin patent. Clowes had a PhD in chemistry and a research interest in cancer. In 1919, he was hired by Eli Lilly Research Laboratory in Indianapolis, Indiana, to monitor academic research for potential new drugs. Today, it is commonplace for pharmaceutical companies and universities to collaborate, but in the 1920s, this was a new idea to which there was still some resistance.

Clowes had been at the 1921 American Physiological Society meeting where Banting had performed so poorly. He saw potential in Banting's research and approached Macleod about cooperating with Lilly, but, at that time, Macleod was not interested. When it became clear that the university's Connaught Laboratory could not keep up with demand, Clowes went to Toronto and tried again. After several visits and some complicated negotiations, he came away with an agreement that gave Eli Lilly exclusive rights to manufacture insulin in the United States.

Initially, Eli Lilly also had trouble scaling up production. Eventually, their head chemist, George Walden (1885–1982) developed a new way of purifying and concentrating insulin that increased both purity and yield. Soon refrigerator cars full of beef and pork pancreases were being delivered to the Indianapolis plant. In 1923, the first year that Eli Lilly made insulin (brand name Iletin) commercially available, they intentionally kept the price low as a goodwill gesture to the public. They still sold $1 million ($14.7 million in 2019 dollars) worth of insulin. Later, the Danish company Nordisk Insulin Laboratory (now Novo Nordisk) acquired the rights to produce insulin for Europe, and Connaught Laboratories continued to supply the drug in Canada.

THE NOBEL PRIZE

In 1923, Frederick Banting and J. J. R. Macleod were jointly awarded the Nobel Prize in Physiology or Medicine, a first for Canada. Banting was furious that Best had been overlooked and that he had to share the prize with Macleod, whom he still believed had stolen credit for his and Best's work. Initially, Banting announced that he would refuse the prize, but he relented, accepted the prize, and split his share of the prize money with Best. Under pressure, Macleod split his prize money with Collip. Banting refused to attend the ceremony in Scandinavia to receive the prize because he did not want to be on the same stage as Macleod. Macleod also declined to attend, feeling it would look bad if he showed up and Banting did not.

THE TEAM BREAKS UP

After the successful development of insulin, Frederick Banting opened a private medical practice in Toronto to treat diabetics. One of his patients was Elizabeth Hughes, the teenager who had spent more than two years on the Allen diet. In Toronto, Banting soon had her eating a 2,200-calorie diet, which is normal for a teenage girl. She sometimes required as many as five insulin shots a day and eventually learned to give the shots to herself. Occasionally she had had dangerous periods of hypoglycemia, but she learned to recognize them and self-treat with sugar. For her, the Allen diet, as strict and painful as it was, had served its purpose and kept her alive until a treatment was found.

Elizabeth Hughes finished high school, went to college, married, and became Elizabeth Hughes Gossett. She had a child and lived to be 74 years old. This was a life she could not have imagined when she was diagnosed with diabetes in 1919.

In addition to his medical practice, Frederick Banting was given a position at the University of Toronto Medical School, was appointed to various medical societies and boards, and received many honors. His research interest shifted to cancer, but, at heart, he was a practicing physician, not a researcher. He also earned a law degree, took up serious painting, and aspired to write his biography.

During World War II, Banting worked with Wilbur Franks at the University of Toronto on the successful development of the antigravity suit, or anti-g suit, worn by aviators and astronauts to prevent them from losing consciousness when exposed to high acceleration forces. He also served as a liaison between British and North American medical services. He was working in this capacity when he was killed in an airplane crash in Gander, Newfoundland, in 1941. He died still believing that Macleod had stolen credit for his work. In 2006, the International Diabetes Foundation and the United Nations declared Banting's birthday, November 14, as World Diabetes Day.

J. J. R. Macleod returned to Scotland, where he became a Regius Professor of Physiology at the University of Aberdeen and was awarded many professional honors. For the remainder of his life, he refused to discuss Banting's charges that he took credit for work that was not his own. He continued to research carbohydrate metabolism, wrote 11 scientific books, and died in 1935 at the age of 59.

Charles Best graduated from medical school. He did postgraduate work in London and then returned to the University of Toronto to head the physiology department after Macleod moved to Scotland. He continued his research on diabetes, for which he received many honors. During World War II, he worked on the Canadian Blood Serum Project, producing dry human blood serum for use by wounded soldiers. After the war, he returned to his lifelong interest in diabetes and died in Toronto in 1978.

James Collip returned to the University of Alberta, where he continued his research into blood chemistry and hormones. He later spent 20 years at McGill University in Montreal, where he supervised an endocrinology laboratory that researched hormones produced by the placenta and the pituitary. He always described himself as being one of the discoverers of insulin, even though he was not included in the Nobel Prize. Surprisingly, given their confrontations during the development of insulin, Collip and Banting became friends. In fact, Banting spent the day before his fatal plane crash visiting Collip in Montreal. Collip ended his academic career as dean of medicine and head of the Department of Medical Research at the University of Western Ontario. He died after a stroke in 1965.

THE ADVANCES CONTINUE

The development of insulin was a lifesaving treatment for diabetics, but because insulin acted rapidly and was effective only for a short time, good glucose control required receiving multiple shots each day. Children sometimes even had to be awakened at night and given insulin to prevent a condition of stunted growth called diabetic dwarfism.

Biochemists soon began experimenting with ways to extend the action of insulin by adding small molecules to the drug. The first commercially available extended-action insulin became available in 1936. Called protamine zinc insulin (PZI), it was made by adding a small protein (protamine) and zinc to insulin. With an extended period of action, the number of daily shots a diabetic needed could be reduced. In some patients, a single shot of PZI could keep glucose levels under control for up to 24 hours. Also in 1936, Sir Harold Percival Himsworth (1905–1993) published a paper distinguishing between two types of diabetes, which he called insulin-sensitive (type 1) and insulin-resistant (type 2). This distinction would prove to have a great impact on how diabetes is treated.

Researchers soon discovered that the length of action of insulin could be changed even more by varying the amount of zinc in the formulation. In 1946, Nordisk Insulin Laboratory introduced an insulin whose action was intermediate to regular insulin and PZI. Over the next 10 years, other formulations with different properties were developed. Researchers also had success in mixing formulations of different-acting insulin in various proportions to control the length of action of the drug. Today, many variations of insulin are available. Some of the current insulin options are discussed in the treatment section of chapter 5.

Synthetic Insulin

Insulin is an evolutionarily old molecule. Even insulin taken from bony fish such as tuna, halibut, bass, or trout will, to some degree, work in humans. Until 1978, all insulin was made from cow or pig pancreases. Thousands of pounds were collected from slaughterhouses daily and sent in refrigerated train cars to factories where insulin was extracted and purified. Beef insulin differs from human insulin by only three amino acids or building blocks. Pork insulin differs by only one amino acid. Still, some people developed undesirable reactions to the drug. In addition, the number of diabetics was growing faster than the supply of animal pancreases. The quest was on to find a way to manufacture a laboratory-produced insulin that was identical to human insulin and to be able to make it in large quantities.

In 1978, David Goeddel (b. 1951) and colleagues at the bio-tech start-up company Genentech created the first synthetic human insulin using recombinant DNA technology. To achieve this, a piece of DNA called a plasmid is removed from an *Escherichia coli* bacterium or yeast cell. A plasmid is a circular piece of DNA found in the cytoplasm of a cell. It can reproduce independently of chromosomes in the nucleus of the cell. Using enzymes, a piece of the plasmid is cut away and replaced with a cloned human gene that controls the production of insulin (a process much more difficult that it sounds). The plasmid with the human gene is then injected into an *E. coli* bacterium or a yeast cell.

The cells with the human gene are grown in a fermentation tank where they rapidly reproduce and begin secreting insulin. When the insulin is harvested and purified, it is structurally identical to human insulin. The first synthetic human insulin, Humulin, was approved in the United States in 1983 and was made by the pharmaceutical company Eli Lilly in cooperation with Genentech.

Insulin Analogs

Research on insulin and the pancreas did not stop with the development of synthetic human insulin. In studying what triggers the release of insulin in healthy individuals, scientists discovered that when blood glucose levels rise, insulin is released from the pancreas in bursts or pulses, not in a steady stream. Scientists felt it would be advantageous to produce a synthetic insulin that more closely mimicked the way the human body works. This led to the development of insulin analogs.

An analog is something that is similar to something else, so insulin analogs are very similar, but not identical to, human insulin. They are constructed by making small changes to the insulin molecule to introduce the desired characteristic. Insulin analogs are injected under the skin rather than into muscle, and, once absorbed, they act like human insulin. The first insulin analog was insulin lispro (brand name Humalog). made by Eli Lilly. It was approved in the United States in 1996. Since then, other insulin analogs have been developed with both short- and long-acting capacity (see chapter 5).

Non-Insulin Drugs

All people with type 1 diabetes need insulin daily, but this is not true of people with type 2 diabetes. Oral medications—that is, drugs taken by mouth—along with a controlled diet and exercise can often keep the blood glucose level of people with type 2 diabetes within safe levels. In medieval times, a plant called goat's rue (*Galega officinalis*) was used in southern Europe as a folk remedy for diabetes. It turns out that this plant contains a chemical that is an antihyperglycemic, or a chemical that lowers blood sugar levels.

In the 1920s, some scientists studied this plant and related chemicals as a treatment for diabetes, but they lost interest when insulin became available. However, renewed interest in this class of chemicals, called biguanides, led to the development of the oral drug metformin. Metformin was approved for use in the United States in 1996. It is usually the first drug prescribed to control blood sugar levels in people with type 2 diabetes. Other oral drugs may also be used by people with type 2 diabetes, depending on how well their diabetes is controlled. Some of these options are discussed in the type 2 treatment section of chapter 5.

Delivery Systems

As new drugs were introduced, new delivery systems were also being developed. In addition to traditional syringe injections, insulin delivery systems now include insulin pens, needleless insulin jet injectors, insulin pumps, and inhaled insulin. Progress has also occurred in tools for home blood glucose testing. A variety of meters are available to analyze glucose in a drop of blood taken from a finger prick. Continuous glucose monitoring by an implantable sensor is also available. These options and their strengths and weaknesses are discussed in the management section of chapter 5.

3

Causes and Risk Factors

As indicated in the first chapter, type 1, type 2, and gestational diabetes are different metabolic disorders that are all related to the body's inability to use glucose for energy. These disorders have substantially different causes and risk factors. Understanding these differences is the key to appropriate treatment as well as expected outcomes. Consequently, each type of diabetes must be considered separately.

TYPE 1 DIABETES

Type 1 diabetes is an autoimmune disease. In an autoimmune disease, the body's immune system malfunctions and destroys healthy body cells. In type 1 diabetes, the cells destroyed are beta cells of the pancreas that produce insulin, the hormone that allows cells to use glucose for energy. Without insulin, glucose cannot enter cells, so it accumulates in the blood. The result is hyperglycemia, which can damage multiple tissues and organs. Meanwhile, the body, desperate for energy, breaks down fat in order to keep functioning. The breakdown of fat results in an increase in the blood level of compounds called ketones. Uncorrected, this leads to a condition called diabetic ketoacidosis (DKA), which is discussed extensively in chapter 5.

A measurement called pH is used to determine the acidity or alkalinity of fluids. The pH of pure water is 7.0. Numbers above this indicate that the fluid is alkaline, while numbers below this indicate that the fluid is acidic (e.g., stomach acid has a pH of about 3.5). The pH of healthy blood is 7.35 or slightly alkaline. Excess ketones in the blood make it more acidic. Ketoacidosis develops when enough ketones decrease the blood pH to 7.30 or lower. Even this relatively small change disrupts blood homeostasis (see chapter 1) and sets off a catastrophic series of chemical events that, without prompt treatment, end in coma and death.

Genetic Factors in Type 1 Diabetes

Type 1 diabetes develops because healthy beta cells are killed, so they no longer produce insulin. Why this happens in some people is not completely clear, but researchers know that genetic factors and the immune system play a role. A properly functioning immune system has built-in controls so that it attacks viruses, foreign bacteria, and abnormal body cells such as cancer cells, but it does not attack healthy body cells.

In an autoimmune disease, these controls fail, and healthy body cells are destroyed. In type 1 diabetes, the immune system attacks beta cells. In other autoimmune diseases, such as multiple sclerosis, rheumatoid arthritis, or celiac disease, other types of healthy cells are attacked. Researchers do not completely understand what triggers the immune system to attack beta cells, but to understand what scientists think may happen, it is necessary to review some basics about the immune system.

Cells and viruses have unique identifying proteins on their surface called antigens. In humans, these proteins are usually referred to as human leukocyte antigens (HLAs). These antigens act as a uniform that says "I belong to this individual." A healthy immune system recognizes the cells, called self cells, that have an individual's proper antigens and leaves them alone. When foreign bacteria or viruses enter the body, they have a different set of antigens on their surfaces. Because their "uniform" is different, immune system cells identify them as nonself cells and attack them.

HLAs on a cell surface are determined by the individual's genetic code. Researchers have identified about two dozen specific gene mutations on chromosome 6 that change the composition of HLA proteins. These specific mutations are found more often in people who develop type 1 diabetes. And yet, not everyone with these mutations develops type 1 diabetes. This suggests that an environmental factor may be involved.

As of 2019, many scientists think that people who have these mutations but are not exposed to a specific environmental trigger continue to produce insulin normally. However, in people who have these mutations and who are exposed to the trigger, the immune system malfunctions and begins to destroy the individual's beta cells. It can take several years to destroy enough beta cells to be noticeable.

When between 80 and 90 percent of beta cells have been killed, the amount of insulin produced is so small that symptoms of diabetes appear. Because the body cannot make more beta cells, insulin deficiency is permanent, and type 1 diabetes becomes a disorder requiring life-long treatment with insulin from an outside source (see chapter 5).

Environmental Factors

As of 2019, the most likely environmental trigger for developing type 1 diabetes in people with certain genetic mutations appears to be infection with a virus. (See chapter 8 for more on how this conclusion was reached.) The most plausible suspects are common viruses that almost everyone is exposed to and that cause familiar symptoms such as fever, sore throat, muscle aches, and diarrhea. The suspect viruses include the mumps virus, Coxsackie B viruses, rotaviruses, cytomegalovirus, and possibly the virus that causes rubella (German measles). These viruses have been found in pancreatic islets that contain beta cells where one would not normally expect to find them. Some researchers have also suggested that exposure to the proteins in cow's milk before the age of three months or exposure to toxic chemicals may be triggers. Nevertheless, viral infections appear to be the most likely environmental trigger in susceptible individuals.

Why do certain viruses act as triggers? Scientists know that some gene mutations common in people with type 1 diabetes but rarely found in the general population change the HLAs on the surface of cells. They believe that these mutations cause the individual's HLAs on beta cells to look abnormal and appear similar to the antigens on the surface of the suspect viruses.

When a person is infected with one of these suspect viruses, immune system cells attack the virus and make antibodies against it to destroy it. Normally these antibodies would not harm self cells. However, because mutations to beta-cell HLAs make the proteins on the surface of the beta cells look similar to the proteins on the surface of the virus, the immune system misidentifies these cells, believes that they are foreign, and continues to make antibodies to kill them. There are many beta cells in the pancreas, and it can take several years for enough of these cells to be killed for type 1 diabetes to become evident. This probably is not the complete story of how type 1 diabetes is caused, but it is the reasoning of many researchers in 2019.

Risk Factors

Most risk factors for developing type 1 diabetes are related to one's genetic inheritance. In identical twins, if one is diagnosed with type 1 diabetes, there is a 50 percent chance the other twin will also develop type 1 diabetes. This compares to about a 5 percent chance that both nonidentical twins will develop the disorder. If a mother has type 1 diabetes, there is a 2 to 3 percent chance that her child will also be affected, but if the father has type 1 diabetes, the risk more than doubles to between 5 and 6 percent. Researchers do not know the reason for this difference. If both parents have type 1 diabetes, the chance of their child developing the disorder is about 30 percent.

Because there is a genetic component to type 1 diabetes, and since ethnic and geographically defined groups are more likely to have children with someone from the same group or region, it follows that the frequency of type 1 diabetes varies considerably around the world. The disorder is most common in Caucasians of northern European ancestry and is highest in Scandinavia. Rates are lowest in China and Japan and are relatively low in people with African ancestry. Geography may also play a role. Type 1 diabetes is more common in cold climates than in warm climates. Some researchers believe this is because people in cold climates spend more time indoors around other people, exposing them to more viral infections that may act as triggers.

People who have another autoimmune disorder are also at higher risk for developing type 1 diabetes. For example, Grave's disease or Hashimoto's thyroiditis, both autoimmune diseases of the thyroid, increase the risk of type 1 diabetes. The frequency of type 1 diabetes is also increased in people with celiac disease, multiple sclerosis, Addison's disease, and many other less common autoimmune disorders.

At one time, young age was considered a risk factor, but this is no longer true. Many people with type 1 diabetes show symptoms and are diagnosed around the age of four. Others show symptoms around puberty, but adults can also develop type 1 diabetes. For example, Jay Cutler, a quarterback who played 12 seasons in the National Football League, was diagnosed at the age of 25 with a form of type 1 diabetes known as latent autoimmune diabetes in adults (LADA), sometimes referred to as type 1.5 diabetes. The Expert Committee on the Diagnosis and Classification of Diabetes Mellitus does not recognize LADA as a separate form of diabetes but considers it a form of type 1 diabetes that develops in adulthood. Adults with LADA are often misdiagnosed as having type 2 diabetes. With a proper diagnosis and the use of an insulin pump, Cutler continued to play professional football for nine seasons after his diagnosis.

TYPE 2 DIABETES

Type 2 diabetes accounts for about 95 percent of all cases of diabetes. Unlike type 1, type 2 diabetes is *not* an autoimmune disease, and it usually does not require treatment with insulin from an outside source (see chapter 5). At one time, type 2 diabetes was thought to be caused only by cellular resistance to insulin. Insulin acts as a key that opens a channel into cells so that glucose can enter and either be used as energy or stored as glucagon (in liver and muscle cells) or as fat (in fat cells). Cells that become insulin resistant are like doors with a broken or sticky lock—hard to open. The glucose channel is no longer easily accessible. The amount of glucose entering insulin-resistant cells decreases, and the amount of glucose in the blood increases, resulting in hyperglycemia.

Hormonal Factors

Originally, insulin resistance was considered the only cause of type 2 diabetes. Researchers now believe that, in addition to insulin resistance, beta cell dysfunction is a factor in who develops the disorder. One reason for this thinking is that almost all obese individuals show insulin resistance, but type 2 diabetes appears to develop only in those people who also have decreased insulin production.

In addition to insulin resistance and decreased insulin production in type 2 diabetes, the reciprocal relationship between glucagon, produced by pancreatic alpha cells (see chapter 1), and insulin, produced by beta cells, is lost. Glucagon produced by alpha cells causes the liver to break down glycogen, a form of stored glucose, and release it into the bloodstream. In a healthy individual, when blood glucose increases after a meal, the amount of insulin secreted by beta cells increases, allowing more glucose to enter cells. At the same time, glucagon production decreases so that the liver does not break down glycogen and release glucose.

As glucose is used by cells and blood glucose levels drop, beta cells decrease the amount of insulin they secrete. When blood glucose levels become low enough, alpha cells sense this and increase their secretion of glucagon. Glucagon stimulates the liver to convert stored glycogen into glucose and release it into the blood. This restores glucose levels to their normal range and maintains homeostasis.

In type 2 diabetes, the balancing act between insulin and glucagon is lost. Inadequate insulin secretion by beta cells, coupled with insulin resistance in body cells, keep glucose levels high. This would normally prevent alpha cells from secreting glucagon, but it does not. Instead, alpha cells act as if glucose levels are too low and secrete glucagon. The liver then pumps more glucose into the blood. where levels are already too high. The result is hyperglycemia, characteristic of type 2 diabetes.

Genetic Factors in Type 2 Diabetes

Genetics, age, and lifestyle choices all play roles in determining who develops type 2 diabetes. It is difficult to determine how much each of these factors contribute. Researchers have found more than a dozen mutations that affect insulin secretion, glucagon secretion, and the ability to sense glucose levels in the blood. They believe that some of these mutations are related to the development of type 2 diabetes. It appears the effect of these mutations is cumulative. In other words, the more of these mutations a person has, the more likely that individual is to develop type 2 diabetes.

The genetic contribution to the development of type 2 diabetes is difficult for researchers to quantify because families share not only genes but often environments and lifestyles. According to the American Diabetes Association (ADA), the overall risk of developing type 2 diabetes is 1 in 7 if one parent was diagnosed with the disorder before the age of 50 and 1 in 13 if one parent was diagnosed after the age 50. If both parents have type 2 diabetes, the risk of their children developing the disorder increases dramatically to one in two, or 50 percent.

Lifestyle and Environmental Risks

Body weight has both a genetic and a lifestyle component, and being overweight or obese is a major risk factor for the development of type 2 diabetes. Overweight is defined as having a body mass index (BMI) of between 25 and 29.9. Obesity is defined as having a BMI of 30 or greater. BMI is the ratio of body weight to height. A BMI calculator can be found at https://www.nhlbi.nih.gov/health/educational/lose_wt/BMI/bmicalc.htm. Although excess weight is a risk factor for type 2 diabetes, not everyone who is overweight or obese develops the disorder. Other factors also increase the risk of developing type 2 diabetes.

• Physical activity level. Physical activity causes cells to use more glucose and appears to reduce insulin resistance. Inactivity appears to increase insulin resistance. People who are physically active fewer than three times a week are at increased risk. The minimum recommended activity for Americans between the ages of 18 and 64 years is

45 minutes five times per week of moderate exercise, such as brisk walking. For Americans over the age of 65, the minimum is 30 minutes five times per week of moderate exercise unless restricted by health or mobility. Exercises to increase strength and improve balance are also recommended.

- Age, race, and culture. The risk of developing type 2 diabetes increases for everyone after they reach the age of 45, but the risk is greater for African Americans, Native Alaskans, Asian Americans, Native Hawaiians, Pacific Islanders, and people of Hispanic/Latino heritage. It is unclear why certain groups have a higher level of risk, but again, a combination of both genetics and lifestyle are thought to play a role.

- Previous gestational diabetes. Women who have had gestational diabetes or given birth to a baby weighing over 9 pounds (4.1 kg) are at higher risk for type 2 diabetes later in life.

- A low level of high-density lipoprotein (HDL) cholesterol, also called "good" cholesterol. This material helps remove fats from the blood.

- A high level of triglycerides, which are fats found in the blood. The healthy level for triglycerides is less than 150 mg/dl (1.7 mmol/L). High levels of triglycerides and low levels of HDL often occur together.

- A history of heart disease or stroke.

- A major depressive disorder or clinical depression.

- Polycystic ovary syndrome. All women produce some male hormones. In polycystic ovary syndrome, a woman produces more male hormones than normal. This causes fluid-filled sacs (cysts) to form in the ovaries, resulting in decreased fertility. Both polycystic ovary syndrome (PCOS) and type 2 diabetes are related to obesity, insulin resistance, and eventually to decreased insulin production, but the mechanisms that control these two disorders are not clear.

- Acanthosis nigricans. This is a condition in which the skin around the neck, armpits, and groin darken. It is a sign of insulin resistance.

- Obstructive sleep apnea. People with obstructive sleep apnea stop breathing for short periods multiple times each night. This condition can cause symptoms unrelated to diabetes, but it has been shown to be more common in people with type 2 diabetes. Both sleep apnea and type 2 diabetes often are obesity related.

- Taking certain prescription drugs. Certain drugs appear to have the potential to accelerate the development of or worsen type 2 diabetes. Although direct cause and effect of these drugs has not been rigorously proven, suspect drugs include diuretics (water pills), glucocorticoid drugs (e.g., cortisone, prednisone), some drugs used to treat chronic obstructive pulmonary disease and chronic asthma, large doses of niacin (also called nicotinic acid), long-term treatment with antibiotics or antiretroviral drugs, and drugs given to prevent the rejection of organ transplants. Individuals with diabetes should check with their physician or pharmacist about potential drug effects on their blood glucose levels.

- Using certain recreational drugs. Regular excessive alcohol consumption is a risk factor for chronic pancreatitis (inflammation of the pancreas). Pancreatitis is a major risk factor for the development of diabetes. Frequent use of opioid drugs also appears to reduce insulin secretion. Amphetamines, methamphetamine, MDMA (ecstasy), and similar stimulant drugs appear to increase the release of chemicals that inhibit insulin production.

Type 2 diabetes is preceded by a condition called prediabetes. In prediabetes, an individual's fasting glucose level is 100–125 mg/dl (5.6–7.0 mmol/L), and the oral glucose test level two hours after drinking a sugary drink is 140–199 mg/dl (7.8–11 mmol/L). These values are above normal but not so high as to allow a diagnosis of diabetes.

The risk factors for prediabetes are the same as for type 2 diabetes. Through changes in diet and increased physical activity, it is possible for people to reverse prediabetes. However, in many people, the condition progresses to type 2 diabetes within five years. The National Institute of Diabetes and Digestive Diseases provides a type 2 diabetes risk assessment questionnaire at https://www.niddk.nih.gov/health-information/diabetes /overview/risk-factors-type-2-diabetes/diabetes-risk-test.

GESTATIONAL DIABETES

Gestational diabetes is a diabetic condition that develops in a pregnant woman who has not previously had diabetes. During pregnancy, the placenta makes hormones that increase insulin resistance. This is normal, but if the body cannot make enough insulin to overcome this increased resistance, gestational diabetes develops. Gestational diabetes occurs in 3–10 percent of pregnancies. Although blood glucose levels drop after the baby is born, some studies have found that women with gestational diabetes have persistent metabolic abnormalities up to three years after their pregnancies and are more likely to develop type 2 diabetes later in life.

Risk factors for developing gestational diabetes include:

- Age, race, and culture. Women over the age of 25 are more likely to develop gestational diabetes. African American, Hispanic, Native American, and Asian women are much more likely to develop gestational diabetes than women of European heritage. About one-third of the women in these high-risk groups will go on to develop type 2 diabetes within five years of delivery.

- Obesity. Most obese individuals have some degree of insulin resistance. Pregnancy tends to increase insulin resistance, leading to hyperglycemia.
- Rapid weight gain during pregnancy.
- Family history. Women with a parent or sibling with type 2 diabetes are more likely to develop gestational diabetes.
- Pregnancy history. Gestational diabetes in a previous pregnancy, having given birth to a baby weighing more than 9 pounds (4.1 kg), or having a stillborn baby increase the rate of gestational diabetes in future pregnancies.
- A diagnosis of prediabetes.
- A diagnosis of polycystic ovary syndrome.

Gestational diabetes usually begins near the start of the third trimester of pregnancy. Women at high risk for gestational diabetes are often tested toward the end of the first trimester, and then again later in pregnancy. Women at average risk are usually tested between weeks 24 and 28 of pregnancy.

Gestational diabetes can increase risks to the fetus, including an increased risk of premature delivery (before 37 weeks) or a late-term stillbirth. Babies born to mothers with gestational diabetes also tend to be large because they share a blood supply with the mother and store extra glucose in the blood as fat. This increases the likelihood of trauma during the birth and may cause the woman's obstetrician to recommend a cesarean birth.

After birth, between 15 and 25 percent of babies born to mothers with gestational diabetes develop hypoglycemia, a condition in which blood glucose drops to unacceptably low levels. While in the womb, the baby overproduced insulin to compensate for the high level of glucose in his or her blood supply. Once the baby is born and no longer shares a blood supply with the mother, there is a period of adjustment before the baby's insulin production returns to normal. If newborn hypoglycemia goes unrecognized, the baby may have seizures; brain damage; coma; and, in extreme cases, may die.

4

Signs and Symptoms

Although the terms sign and symptom are often used interchangeably, there is a difference. Symptoms are subjective feelings the individual experiences. These include sensations such as pain, anxiety, dizziness, nausea, headache, ringing in the ears, fatigue, or blurred vision. Signs are objective abnormalities that are visible to other people and can often be measured. Examples of signs are sweating, abnormal blood pressure, elevated temperature, pallor, joint swelling, and difficulty breathing. Signs also include the results of tests, such as a complete blood count, urinalysis, x-rays, or microscopic examination of tissue samples.

Sometimes signs and symptoms guide physicians to order specific tests for diabetes, such as fasting glucose test, oral glucose test, and urinalysis. More often, symptoms of type 1 diabetes go unrecognized, especially in children, until a large percentage of beta cells have been destroyed. Then symptoms suddenly worsen and cannot be ignored.

In type 2 diabetes, symptoms tend to be vague. Since these symptoms may not cause pain or interfere with daily life, people often dismiss them as unimportant or as minor annoyances. This explains why in 2017, about 7.2 million Americans had type 2 diabetes but remained undiagnosed. Worldwide, the International Diabetes Foundation estimates that half of all people with type 2 diabetes remain undiagnosed and untreated, either through lack of access to health care or because symptoms are unrecognized or attributed to natural aging. In these situations, diabetes is often first diagnosed during a visit to the doctor for another problem, such as slow wound healing, failing vision, or one of the many other complications diabetes quietly causes. Tests used to diagnose diabetes are covered in chapter 5, and complications are discussed in chapter 6.

TYPE 1 DIABETES

The classic symptoms of type 1 diabetes are excessive thirst, excessive urination, excessive hunger, and unexplained weight loss. Excessive thirst (polydipsia) occurs due to excess glucose in the blood, or hyperglycemia. Normally, a part of the kidney (the glomerulus) filters out glucose, small molecules, and water from the blood. Useful substances are reabsorbed into the bloodstream in another part of the kidney (the tubules), while waste products from cellular metabolism, along with excess water, are removed from the body in urine. In a healthy person, all the filtered glucose is reabsorbed.

When glucose builds up in the blood to around 200 ml/dL (11.1 mg/dl) and stays there, the kidneys can no longer reabsorb all the glucose that was filtered out. Glucose remains in the tubules and is excreted in urine. The urine may smell or taste sweet because of the glucose it contains. This sweet urine, a condition now called glycosuria, was one of the first signs of diabetes that doctors recognized in ancient times. The glucose that remains in the tubules drags water with it that would normally be reabsorbed. The loss of this extra water upsets fluid balance in the body. This causes a person to feel thirsty and drink more water.

Drinking more water causes the second symptom of diabetes, excessive urination (polyuria). At first, drinking more and urinating more keep the amount of fluid in the body more or less in balance. Nevertheless, as the disorder progresses, hyperglycemia increases, and more and more glucose is filtered into the tubules. More water is required to dilute this glucose. Eventually, more water is excreted as urine than the individual drinks. This results in dehydration.

Dehydration produces some of the more general symptoms of diabetes, including headache, nausea, and dizziness. As dehydration continues, the kidneys work to retain water that the body needs by creating less urine. This requires the kidneys to work harder and can result in kidney damage. Also, in response to prolonged dehydration, the body produces hormones that interfere with the action of insulin. These hormones, in conjunction with reduced urine production, accelerate the rise in blood glucose levels. Blurred vision, another symptom of diabetes, can also occur from dehydration, as water is pulled out of the tissues of the eye.

Excessive hunger (polyphagia) and unintended weight loss occur because cells are starved for glucose. A person with type 1 diabetes may be eating enough calories, but, in the absence of adequate insulin (remember, in type 1 diabetes, beta cells that make insulin are destroyed), the glucose produced by digestion of the food a person eats cannot enter cells. In response to glucose starvation in the cells, the body breaks down muscle and fat to provide more glucose. This can cause fatigue, muscle weakness, and weight loss, but, more seriously, it can lead to diabetic ketoacidosis (DKA). DKA is a medical emergency. It develops as a side effect of the body breaking down large amounts of fat for energy. When fat is broken down, breakdown products called ketones increase the acidity of the blood. Even small increases in blood acidity set off cascading effects that can end in coma or death. DKA is discussed more extensively in chapter 5.

Signs of type 1 diabetes often seem to appear suddenly, although the destruction of beta cells and the decrease in insulin production has usually been progressing for a year or more. These symptoms are often missed, especially in children. For many people with type 1 diabetes, DKA is the first sign that they have the disorder. DKA can be reversed with prompt medical treatment, but it can be fatal if not treated promptly.

TYPE 2 DIABETES

Type 2 diabetes is usually preceded by a condition called prediabetes, also known as intermediate hyperglycemia. Tests show that people with prediabetes have glucose levels that are higher than normal, but they are not high enough to be considered diabetes. Prediabetes can often be reversed by changes in diet and increased physical activity; however, the American Diabetes Association (ADA) estimates that about 70 percent of people with prediabetes go on to develop type 2 diabetes. This is partly because prediabetes has few symptoms. Most people, unless they are specifically tested for glucose tolerance, simply do not know that they have prediabetes and are at risk for developing type 2 diabetes.

Prediabetes diabetes progresses to type 2 diabetes gradually, and again, many people fail to recognize that their symptoms indicate diabetes. Most symptoms of type 2 diabetes are the same as for type 1 diabetes—increased thirst, increased urination, and increased hunger. Since people with type 2 diabetes continue to produce some insulin, there is less weight loss than in type 1 diabetes. Most people with type 2 diabetes are overweight or obese, so any loss may go unnoticed. People with type 2 diabetes may blame stress for unusual fatigue and natural aging for changes in urination and vision.

It is possible for DKA to be the first recognized symptom of type 2 diabetes, but this is unusual.

Over time, serious complications of type 2 diabetes can develop. These complications are discussed extensively in chapter 6. Complications that occur early in the progress of the disorder are often the first symptoms for which an individual seeks medical advice. Tingling or a pins-and-needles sensation (paresthesia) in the hands and feet and/or a burning pain in the arms, hands, legs, or feet are early indications of peripheral nerve damage that can be caused by diabetes. In addition, diabetes reduces the body's ability to fight infection. Gums may become sore and swollen, and pockets of pus can develop between the gums and the teeth. Of those people with gum disease, 90 percent are at high risk for developing type 2 diabetes. In addition, genital yeast infections that cause itching and discharge in women and swelling of the head of the penis, redness, discharge, itchiness, and pain (a condition called balanitis) may occur in men. Men may also experience erectile dysfunction, especially if their diabetes has gone untreated for a long time. Although these conditions have other causes, undiagnosed type 2 diabetes is often the cause.

GESTATIONAL DIABETES

Gestational diabetes usually causes no symptoms. Women at high risk for gestational diabetes (see chapter 3) are given a fasting glucose test during the first trimester of pregnancy and again later in pregnancy. Women at low risk are usually given the same test between weeks 24 and 28 of pregnancy.

Overall, the symptoms of all types of diabetes frequently go unrecognized because they are general (e.g., fatigue, nausea) and are common to other disorders. The sign of diabetes—that is hyperglycemia—is easily determined and definitive, but it is detected only if the physician orders the appropriate tests. These diagnostic tests are discussed in the next chapter.

5

Diagnosis, Treatment, and Management

Diagnosing diabetes is usually straightforward. Definitive diagnosis can be obtained by testing the level of glucose in the blood. Once certain tests indicate that the blood glucose level is higher than 126 mg/dl (7.0 mmol/L), the individual is diagnosed as diabetic. In rare circumstances, additional tests are needed to distinguish between type 1 and type 2 diabetes.

DIAGNOSTIC TESTS

Many cases of type 2 and gestational diabetes produce no symptoms and go unrecognized by the individual. For that reason, the American Diabetes Association (ADA) recommends regular blood glucose tests for people in the following groups, even when an individual is symptom free:

• Asian Americans whose BMI is greater than 23, and anyone else with a BMI greater than 25 who has any additional risk factors should be tested regardless of age. (See chapter 3, "Lifestyle and Environmental Risks" for an explanation of BMI and risk factors.)

• Anyone over the age of 45 should be tested, with the test repeated every three years if results are normal.

- Anyone who has been diagnosed with prediabetes should be tested yearly.
- Any woman who has had gestational diabetes should be tested every three years and early in subsequent pregnancies.

Fasting Blood Glucose Test

A fasting blood glucose test requires that the individual eat or drink nothing except water for at least eight hours before the test. To perform the test, a blood sample is drawn either from a vein or a finger prick. A normal result is a blood glucose level of less than 100 mg/dl (5.6 mmol/L). A reading of 100–125 mg/dl (5.6–7.0 mmol/L) indicates prediabetes, and a reading greater than 126 mg/dl (7.0 mmol/L) results in a diagnosis of diabetes. Fasting blood tests are generally fast and accurate. However, some common medications can affect glucose levels. These include antipsychotics, aspirin, birth control pills, diuretics, monoamine oxidase inhibitors, some antidepressant medications, and steroid drugs. People being tested should review their medications and supplements with their physicians to assure proper interpretation of the results. Recent heart attack, severe stress, surgery, or trauma can also alter results.

Random Glucose Test

A random glucose test is done in the same way as a fasting glucose test, only the individual may eat at any time before the test. This is not a definitive diagnostic test. Any reading higher than 200 mg/dl (11 mmol/L) suggests diabetes and requires additional testing.

Oral Glucose Tolerance Test

The oral glucose tolerance test (OGTT) can be used to screen for type 2 diabetes or gestational diabetes. This test is not used to detect type 1 diabetes. The test measures how easily glucose enters cells. A one-step approach is used to test for type 2 diabetes, while a two-step test is used to test for gestational diabetes. To prepare, the individual eats or drinks nothing for at least eight hours before the test. At the start of the test, blood is drawn to determine the fasting blood glucose level. The individual then drinks a solution containing 72 grams (2.6 oz) of sugar. A blood sample is taken two hours after drinking the sugar solution. A reading of 140–199 mg/dl

(7.8–11 mmol/L) at the two-hour mark indicates prediabetes, and a reading of 200 mg/dl (11.1 mmol/L) or higher triggers a diabetes diagnosis.

An OGTT is routinely used to screen for gestational diabetes between weeks 24 and 28 of pregnancy, or earlier if the woman is considered at high risk for hyperglycemia. The ADA recommends a modified version of the procedure described above for diagnosing gestational diabetes, with different glucose values indicating diabetes in pregnancy. In this two-hour test, blood is first drawn while fasting, again at one hour, and then again at two hours. Readings greater than 91 mg/dl (5.1 mmol/L) fasting, 179 mg/dl (9.9 mmol/L) at one hour, and 152 mg/dl (8.4 mmol/L) at two hours indicate gestational diabetes. Only one timed reading needs to exceed the threshold for gestational diabetes to be diagnosed. The American College of Obstetricians and Gynecologists recommends a three-hour test using a 100-gram (3.5 oz) sugar solution, with blood drawn at hourly intervals for three hours and slightly different glucose readings to indicate diabetes.

Glycated Hemoglobin (A1c) Test

An A1c test, sometimes called a glycated hemoglobin (HbA1c) test, can be used to help diagnose and manage prediabetes and type 2 diabetes, but it is not usually considered a definitive diagnostic test for either disorder. The A1c test cannot be used to diagnose type 1 diabetes, gestational diabetes, or cystic fibrosis–related diabetes, although it can be used as a tool in the management of these disorders.

The A1c test measures the average blood glucose level over the preceding three months. The test is based on the fact that glucose binds with hemoglobin, the molecule in red blood cells that carries oxygen around the body. The higher the glucose level in the blood, the greater the amount of glucose that will bind with hemoglobin, and the higher the A1c value. The test measures a three-month average glucose level, because three months is the approximate life span of a red blood cell.

Blood can be drawn for an A1c test at any time of day; the individual does not have to be fasting. A1c results are as follows: normal—less that 5.7 percent; prediabetes—5.7 to 6.4 percent; diabetes—greater than 6.4 percent. Various conditions can affect the accuracy of an A1c test, including sickle cell disease, recent blood loss, hemodialysis, blood transfusion, iron-deficiency anemia, kidney failure, or liver disease. After a high A1c test, diagnosis of type 2 diabetes is normally confirmed by an OGTT. Once diabetes is established, A1c testing is used as a management tool. Table 5.1 shows the correlation between A1c values and the three-month average blood glucose level.

Table 5.1   Relationship of A1c to Average Blood Glucose Level

A1c	mg/dl	mmol/L
5%	90	5.0
5.5%	111	5.5
6%	126	7.0
6.5%	140	7.8
7%	154	8.6
7.5	169	9.4
8%	183	10.1
8.5%	197	10.9
9%	212	11.8
9.5%	226	12.6
10%	240	13.4

Source: American Diabetes Association. 2019. https://professional.diabetes.org/diapro/glucose_calc.

Antibody Testing

Usually the kind of diabetes—type 1 or type 2—is easy to distinguish, although some unusual variants, such as LADA, monogenic diabetes, and cystic fibrosis–related diabetes may initially cause confusion. When a patient does not respond to treatment as expected, the initial diagnosis as to type must be reconsidered and additional tests performed. These are specialized tests that are not used for routine diagnosis.

The C-peptide test measures how much C-peptide protein is in the blood. The amount of this protein correlates to the amount of insulin the body is producing. Absent or very low levels of C-peptide indicate type 1 diabetes.

Some tests measure the presence of specific antibodies in the blood. Because type 1 diabetes is an autoimmune disease, the body makes antibodies that destroy beta cells in the pancreas. In type 2 diabetes, insulin production is reduced, but beta cells are not destroyed; thus, there are no beta-cell-destroying antibodies in the blood. Five tests for antibodies may be used to distinguish type 1 from type 2 diabetes. Often more than one test is used because there can be false negatives. These specialized tests are as follows:

- Insulin Autoantibodies (IAA) checks for antibodies against insulin.
- Glutamic Acid Decarboxylase Autoantibodies (GADA) checks for antibodies made against an enzyme that beta cells make only when they form insulin.

- Insulinoma Associated-2-Autoantibodies (IA-2A) checks for antibodies against a different enzyme made by pancreatic cells.

- Zinc Transporter-8 Autoantibodies (ZnT8A), a relatively new test, looks for antibodies against another enzyme that beta cells make when producing insulin.

- Islet Cell Cytoplasmic Autoantibodies (ICA), an older, rarely used test, looks at the reaction between the patient's islet cells and proteins from an animal pancreas.

TYPE 1 DIABETES INITIAL TREATMENT

Diabetic ketoacidosis (DKA) is a complication of diabetes. It can occur any time a person with insulin-dependent diabetes is deprived of adequate insulin. It is discussed here under initial treatment because for as many as one-third of children with type 1 diabetes, DKA is the first indication that they are diabetic. The condition must be reversed before ongoing management of diabetes can begin.

DKA is a state of severe uncontrolled diabetes that is a life-threatening emergency. Although it can occasionally occur in people with type 2 diabetes, it is most common in people with type 1 diabetes. DKA occurs when there is not enough insulin in the body. Inadequate insulin can result from undiagnosed diabetes, infections or illnesses that cause changes in body metabolism, skipping insulin doses, miscalculating insulin dosage, mechanical failure of an insulin pump (see "Insulin Delivery Systems," below), alcohol or drug abuse, heart attack, physical trauma, or severe emotional trauma.

When too little or no insulin is present, glucose levels in the blood increase dramatically (hyperglycemia), while the body starves because glucose cannot enter cells. The body responds to starvation in several ways. The liver breaks down glycogen into glucose and pumps it into the bloodstream because cells are starving. This increases hyperglycemia, because this extra glucose cannot enter cells.

As cells continue to starve, stored fat is broken down into fatty acids as an alternative source of energy. When fatty acids are used by cells, they produce waste products called ketones and ketoacids. These compounds enter the bloodstream and make the blood more acidic. The body tries to get rid of ketones and excess glucose through increased urine production. This causes severe dehydration and the loss in urine of vital electrolytes such as potassium (K^+), sodium (Na^+), and chloride (Cl^-). These electrolytes must stay in balance in order for heart, muscle, and nerve cells to function properly.

When blood homeostasis is disrupted (for more on homeostasis, see chapter 1, "Blood Glucose Regulation"), symptoms of DKA can appear in less than 24 hours. These include a general feeling of weakness and exhaustion; nausea and vomiting; increased urine output, with glucose and ketones in the urine; decreased perspiration; and rapid breathing. The individual's breath may smell like nail polish remover or acetone from ketones in exhaled air. Symptoms are often accompanied by disorientation, confusion, and sometimes coma. Left untreated, the individual will die. DKA is the leading cause of death in children and adolescents with type 1 diabetes.

Almost all children and most adults who arrive at the emergency room with DKA require treatment in an intensive care unit (ICU) and a stay of several days in the hospital to be stabilized. Treatment consists of rapid- and short-acting insulin; intravenous fluid and electrolyte replacement; and treatment with an alkaline compound, such as sodium bicarbonate, to help neutralize acid in the blood. In addition, any illness or infection that triggered DKA is treated. Once the individual is stabilized, diabetes education and long-term management can begin.

Management Requirements

People with type 1 diabetes can do whatever people without the disorder can do. The only difference is that they must be more careful about what they eat and balance their diet and activity level with the proper insulin dosage. Some famous people who have lived for years with type 1 diabetes include Supreme Court Justice Sonia Sotomayor, who was diagnosed with type 1 diabetes at the age of eight; Olympic gold-medalist swimmer Gary Hall, Jr.; Chris Dudley, who played basketball in the NBA for 16 years; Kyle Cochran, a finalist on the television show *American Ninja Warrior*; and Sam Talbot, celebrity chef. What these people have in common with anyone with type 1 diabetes is that they must, under medical direction, take responsibility for understanding and controlling the disorder for the remainder of their lives.

Management of type 1 diabetes is individualized and changes over time as age, activity level, diet, and health status change. Good management requires frequent glucose testing, carbohydrate counting, and adjustments in insulin dosage in order to keep blood glucose levels in the near-normal range. Poor glucose regulation leads to serious complications and often a shortened life span. These complications are discussed in chapter 6.

Successful management is heavily dependent on the individual's compliance with medication administration, dietary restrictions, and testing. Teens, for example, often go through a stage where they resist the dietary and testing requirements needed to control the disorder. For young children with type 1 diabetes, management is a family affair, with much of the responsibility falling on parents and guardians. The responsibility can be overwhelming at first. Certified diabetes educators are invaluable in helping newly-diagnosed patients and their families cope with the demands of managing the disorder.

Management Goals for Type 1 Diabetes

Managing type 1 diabetes requires a team, especially when the individual is a child. At the center of the team are the child or teenager and family members who are in direct contact with the child's physician, diabetes educator, nurse, dietitian, and often a social worker. Other people may be involved in a less direct way, including school personnel, childcare providers, and sports coaches who need to be educated about the disorder. Community support groups for diabetics may benefit both children and their caregivers.

The overall management goal for people with diabetes is to keep the blood glucose level as close to normal as possible and to avoid high and low swings in blood sugar. General recommendations of the ADA for adults aged 18 to 65 years old are shown in Table 5.2. These are only guidelines. Individual target goals are set in consultation with a physician and the diabetes team and may change over time. For example, children under the age of 18 and adults over the age of 65 may have an A1c target of 7.5 percent, while adults over the age of 65 with some health problems may have a target A1c of less than 8.0 percent, and those over the age of 65 with serious health problems may have a target of less than 8.5 percent. The target A1c is also affected by whether the individual is taking drugs that cause hypoglycemia and whether he or she has had any hypoglycemic incidents. Especially among the elderly, hypoglycemia can cause dizziness and increase the risk of falls, which gerontologists point out can be more harmful to health than a slightly higher A1c.

Hypoglycemia

Most people with type 1 diabetes have episodes of hypoglycemia, or low blood sugar. Hypoglycemia can be caused by too much insulin, too little food, too much unplanned physical activity, illness, or some combination of these events. Episodes of hypoglycemia are especially common in young children during the night. Before the development of the first long-acting insulin in 1936, parents had to wake children during the night for an insulin injection to prevent hypoglycemic episodes. Children who were not given this middle-of-the-night shot often developed an enlarged liver and stunted growth, a condition known as diabetic dwarfism.

Table 5.2   Glucose Guidelines for Adults Aged 18–65 Years

Measurement	Person without Diabetes	Person with Diabetes
A1c	< 5.7%	< 7.0%*
Glucose level before meal	< 70–99 mg/dl (3.9–5.5 mmol/L)	80–130 mg/dl (4.4–7.2 mmol/L)
Glucose level 2 hours after meal	< 140 mg/dl (7.8 mmol/L)	< 180 mg/dl (10.0 mmol/L)

*See Chapter 9 Medical Controversies.

Older children and adults usually learn to recognize feelings that indicate their blood glucose is too low and can take prompt corrective action. Adults who spend time with young children who are diagnosed with diabetes need to be aware of the signs of falling glucose levels, because children may not be able to articulate what they are feeling. Glucose levels should be checked immediately whenever hypoglycemia is suspected.

There are three levels of hypoglycemia.

- Level 1: glucose level < 70 mg/dl (3.9 mmol/L). The individual often feels shaky, cold, sweaty, and becomes pale. This requires treatment with a fast-acting carbohydrate, such as fruit juice, a regular (not diet) soft drink, honey, hard candy, or glucose tablets, with a recheck of blood glucose levels in 15 minutes.

- Level 2: glucose level < 54 mg/dl (3.0 mmol/L). The individual shows level 1 symptoms and may also have dizziness, nausea, tingling of the lips and tongue, a fast heartbeat, and mood changes. Treatment is the same as for level 1 hypoglycemia.

- Level 3: glucose level very low, but not specifically defined. The individual may have slurred speech, confusion, staggering gate, convulsions, lose consciousness, or be difficult to wake up. Sometimes severe hypoglycemia in adults is mistaken for drunkenness.

Preventing hypoglycemic episodes is considered more important than meeting the absolute guidelines in Table 5.2. Consequently, some physicians prefer to keep target blood glucose levels slightly higher than the recommended guidelines.

Insulin

Insulin is an evolutionarily ancient molecule. J. J. R. Macleod, cowinner of the Nobel Prize for the discovery of insulin (see chapter 2) tried extracting insulin from bony fish and discovered that it lowered blood sugar in humans, although not as effectively and with more side effects than insulin from pork or beef pancreas.

Before the discovery of insulin in 1922, most children died within one year of diagnosis. The rare adult who developed type 1 diabetes did not live much longer. Between 1922 and 1983, all insulin was extracted from pork or beef pancreases collected from slaughterhouses in huge quantities and shipped under refrigeration to pharmaceutical manufacturing plants. The chemical structure of this animal insulin is very similar to that of human insulin. In 1983, the United States Food and Drug Administration (FDA) approved the first bioengineered synthetic human insulin for use in the United States. Today, all insulin in the United States comes from synthetic sources (see chapter 2, "Synthetic Insulin"), although animal insulin is still available in a few countries.

Synthetic human insulin has several advantages. It eliminates negative side effects some people develop from injecting pork or beef insulin, and it is acceptable to vegetarians, vegans, and those who do not eat pork because it is not an animal product. In addition, pharmaceutical companies no longer have to adjust to seasonal variations in the number of animal pancreases available; they can produce a steady amount of insulin year-round. The three major manufacturers of insulin are Eli Lilly, based in the United States; Novo Nordisk, based in Denmark; and Sanofi, based in France.

All Insulin Is Not Alike

Many variants of synthetic human insulin have been developed and continue to be created. These variants, called insulin analogs, change the time it takes for insulin to lower blood glucose levels and vary the length of time the drug remains effective. Insulin analogs are injected under the skin just like regular synthetic insulin, but they contain small structural changes that alter the rate at which they are used by the body. More than 20 different insulin analogs are available in the United States.

Insulin is also manufactured in different strengths. Insulin concentration is measured in USP Insulin Units (U). Individual doses are calculated by the number of units needed. The most common concentration is U-100. This means that there are 100 units of insulin in 1 milliliter of solution. U-100 is available worldwide. Higher concentrations of insulin, such as U-200 (200 U/ml), U-300 (300 U/ml), and U-500 (500 U/ml) are available in the United States. Availability of these higher concentration insulins varies from country to country. Diabetics traveling outside their home countries should be alert to these variations. A lower concentration, U-40, is available in some countries. In the United States, U-40 is used only in veterinary medicine, mostly to treat older dogs and cats. About 1 percent of dogs who reach 12 years of age develop diabetes, and about one in 230 cats develop the disorder during their lifetimes.

Except for inhaled insulin, which is not widely used, insulin is injected subcutaneously—that is under the skin but not into the muscle. Insulin injected into muscle may be used too quickly, resulting in hypoglycemia. Insulin cannot be taken by mouth because stomach acids will inactivate it, although researchers are working on an oral delivery method (see chapter 10).

The insulin regimen is always individualized and may change frequently to adjust to variations in exercise, diet, and illness. Three aspects to consider in developing an insulin regimen are the speed at which the insulin is absorbed and begins to work (onset), the time at which the insulin is most effective (peak of action), and the length of time the insulin remains effective (duration). Most regimens consist of several the different types of insulin. Optimal glucose control can require injections two, three, or multiple times each day. Table 5.3 summarizes the onset, peak of action, and duration of different types of insulin.

A combination of insulin and insulin analogs is given at different times of day to best mimic the way the body normally produces insulin in response to the individual's activity level, food intake, and health status. Figuring out the dosage and timing requirements can be complex and may change frequently, even daily if, for example, the individual works out at the gym or has sports competition on some days but not others. However, the goal is always to create a regimen that keeps blood glucose near normal levels.

Most regimens for type 1 diabetes call for basal doses of longer duration insulin to keep some baseline level of insulin in the body. These doses are known as basal doses. Extra doses of more rapid-acting insulin are usually given shortly before meals. These are known as bolus doses. Additional insulin and/or food may be needed before bedtime to prevent nighttime or early morning hypo- or hyperglycemia. Consultations with a doctor and diabetes educator are essential in determining the appropriate regimen. It takes some experimentation for newly diagnosed individuals to develop an effective insulin plan. With experience, people with diabetes learn to make adjustments on their own based on blood glucose monitoring, activity level, diet, and experience with different types of insulin.

Counting Carbohydrates

The body needs glucose, and almost all glucose comes from the breakdown of sugar and complex carbohydrates that are found in starchy foods, such as pasta, bread, cereal, corn, rice, lentils, and dried beans. All fruits

Table 5.3   Insulin Types and Their Actions

Type of Insulin	Average Time to Onset	Peak of Action	Approximate Duration	Generic Names	U.S. Brand Names
Rapid-acting	5–10 minutes	1–2 hours	3–4 hours	insulin aspart	NovoLog
				insulin glulisine	Apidra
				insulin lispro	Humalog
Rapid-acting inhaled	5–15 minutes	30–60 minutes	2–3 hours	insulin inhalation	Afrezza
Short-acting or regular	30–60 minutes	2–3 hours	3–6 hours	regular insulin	Humulin R Novolin R
Intermediate-acting	2–4 hours	4–12 hours	12–18 hours	neutral protamine Hagedorn (NPH) or isophane	Humulin N Novolin N
Long-acting	1–2 hours	fairly constant; no peak	20–26 hours	insulin detemir insulin glargine	Levemir Lantus and Basaglar
Ultra-long-acting	6 hours	fairly constant; no peak	36 hours	insulin glargine U-300	Toujeo
	1–2 hours	fairly constant; no peak	44 hours	degludec	Trebisa

contain sugar, as do some vegetables, such as carrots, peas, squash, tomatoes, and turnips. Milk, yogurt, and soy beverages contain some carbohydrates, and cake, candy, chocolate, fruit juice, and regular (not diet) soft drinks contain a lot of sugar. Therefore, what a person with diabetes eats has a great effect on the amount of insulin he or she needs.

To figure out how much insulin will keep blood glucose levels in the target range after each meal, the diabetic individual must know two things. The first is his or her personal insulin-to-carbohydrate (I:C) ratio. The second is the amount of carbohydrates in the food to be consumed.

The I:C ratio is the amount of carbohydrate in grams (g) that one unit of fast-acting insulin will cover or allow the body to use. This ratio is used to calculate the bolus dose, or dose of insulin given all at once before meals, that will keep blood glucose levels within a safe range. The I:C ratio differs for each person and is determined by the diabetic team. Generally, the ratio falls between 1:10 and 1:20. If, for example, a person's I:C ratio is 1:15, one unit of fast-acting insulin is needed for every 15 g of carbohydrates eaten. If the I:C is 1:10, the individual will need one unit of fast-acting insulin for every 10 grams of carbohydrates he or she eats.

If a child with an I:C of 1:15 eats a sandwich made with two slices of bread, each containing 15 g of carbohydrates and meat (which contains very few carbohydrates and is not counted), the child consumes 30 g of carbohydrates and needs two units of fast-acting insulin to metabolize the meal. If the child drinks one cup of milk with lunch, that adds another 15 g of carbohydrates, so three units of insulin are needed to cover the meal. Too much insulin, and the child may develop hypoglycemia. Too little, and hyperglycemia will occur.

Calculating the amount of insulin to take before a meal or snack requires knowing the amount of carbohydrates in the food and the portion or serving size. The best source of this information is a food nutrition label, where both the serving size and the amount of carbohydrates per serving are listed. There are also free smartphone apps to look up this information when food labels are not available. Other useful smartphone apps can track carbohydrate consumption for an entire day.

In the United States and Canada, food labels list total carbohydrates and fiber separately. Fiber is a form of carbohydrate that does not break down in the body, so it does not need to be covered by insulin. To accurately calculate the amount of carbohydrates that insulin must cover from food labels in these two countries, the grams of fiber per serving are subtracted from the total carbohydrates per serving, and that number is used in the I:C calculation. In the United Kingdom, the sugar content per serving is listed on food labels, but fiber is not listed. In doing the I:C calculation in the United Kingdom, the number of grams of sugar are used for the I:C the calculation.

Matching the bolus dose of insulin to the meal to be eaten also requires food be measured. Table 5.4 lists the portion sizes of some common foods that contain 15 g of carbohydrates.

The speed at which glucose levels rise after eating is affected by the type of food, as well as the carbohydrate content. Fruit juice and regular soft drinks cause the largest and most rapid rise in blood glucose, which is why they are often given to combat hypoglycemia. Sugar in fruits such as oranges and apples also promptly raise blood glucose, although not as fast as fruit juice. In addition, carbohydrates eaten with a meal that is heavy in fats and protein are absorbed more slowly than when they are eaten alone. Balancing insulin requirements against food eaten is challenging, although most people find it becomes easier with experience. The best sources of help are

Table 5.4   Food Portions Equaling 15 Grams of Carbohydrates

Food	Serving Size
Apple	1 small
Banana	1 extra small
Orange	1 medium
Fruit juice	½ cup (125 ml)
Raisins	2 tablespoons
Milk	1 cup (250 ml)
Soy beverages, unsweetened	1 cup (250 ml)
Oatmeal, cooked	½ cup (125 ml)
Pasta, cooked	½ cup (125 ml)
Rice, brown or white, cooked	⅓ cup (75 ml)
Potato, boiled or mashed	½ cup (250 ml)
Corn	½ cup (250 ml)
Peas	½ cup (250 ml)
Ice cream	½ cup (250 ml)

dietitians experienced in working with diabetics and diabetes educators. They can also recommend smartphone apps that can simplify calculations.

Alcohol

Alcohol consumption requires special consideration because alcohol can lower blood glucose levels so that the individual who is drinking may require less insulin than usual. When blood glucose is low, the liver breaks down glycogen into glucose to keep blood glucose levels stable. Alcohol blocks the liver from doing this, so there is no backup system for raising blood glucose levels when a person drinks alcohol. This can cause the individual to become hypoglycemic. Alcohol can affect blood glucose levels for more than 24 hours. Blood glucose levels should be checked before drinking alcohol, during drinking, and before bed after drinking.

The ADA recommends that men with type 1 diabetes have no more than two alcoholic drinks within a 24-hour period and women no more than one. A single drink is defined as a 12-ounce beer, a 5-ounce glass of wine, or 1½ ounces of distilled spirits (vodka, whiskey, gin, rum, etc.). The ADA also suggests that people eat something containing carbohydrates while they drink to help prevent hypoglycemia. They recommend that individuals experiment with alcohol consumption at home or in a safe environment until they know how their bodies react and to always wear an identification bracelet that indicates they have diabetes. In addition, anyone with diabetes who staggers, develops slurred speech, or vomits after drinking alcohol should be taken to the emergency room, as this may be a sign of life-threatening hypoglycemia and not just a sign of overconsumption of alcohol.

Blood Glucose Monitoring

The key to preventing complications from diabetes is to keep blood glucose levels as close as possible to the normal range. This requires frequent monitoring. Before the late 1970s, the only way to monitor glucose levels was to test for glucose that spilled over into urine when blood glucose rose too high. This was not a very accurate or efficient way of monitoring glucose levels, because it informed the individual only after glucose levels were too high. It did not provide information that allowed the diabetic to take steps to prevent hyperglycemia from developing.

Monitors that allow personal home testing of blood glucose came into common use in the early 1980s. They require three items: a glucose meter, test strips, and a lancet. With home testing, frequent monitoring of blood glucose became easier and more accurate. Diabetics could see whether their blood glucose was rising or falling and make corrections in diet and medication as needed.

Most people with type 1 diabetes must monitor their blood glucose level at least four times a day—before each meal and at bedtime. Almost all newly diagnosed individuals and many people who have been managing their diabetes for a longer time must check more often, sometimes as often as 10 (yes, 10!) times each day to achieve good glucose control. In addition to before-meal and bedtime testing, they may need to test at a specific interval after eating, before and after exercising, if they wake up at night, when the first get up in the morning, and whenever they begin to feel shaky or hypoglycemic. The frequency of testing becomes even more important when they are ill.

Managing glucose levels on sick days is challenging. The chemicals released to fight illness can interfere with the action of insulin, causing glucose levels to rise. In many cases, insulin dosage must be increased during illness. On the other hand, illness that causes nausea, vomiting, diarrhea, or otherwise interferes with eating can cause insufficient food intake and dehydration. In these situations, hypoglycemia can develop.

On sick days, the general recommendation is to test blood glucose levels every two to three hours and to test for ketones in urine every four hours (see "Ketone Testing," below). Sick individuals should seek medical advice promptly when glucose levels are excessively high or low or ketones are high. Any signs of DKA, as described earlier in this chapter, indicate a medical emergency. Frequent glucose testing is one of the more burdensome aspects of diabetes, but it gives the individual the tools to achieve the good glucose control essential to preventing the serious complications discussed in chapter 6.

Standard Glucose Meters

Glucose meters can be divided into two types: standard glucose meters and continuous glucose meters (CGMs). Standard glucose meters are used with test strips and a lancet, or piercing device (see below). A drop of blood is placed on a test strip that is inserted into the meter. The meter reads the amount of glucose in the blood and shows the result on a screen. The reading is a snapshot of blood glucose at the time the sample is taken.

Many models of glucose meters are available at a variety of price points. All meters are not equally accurate. In the United States, the FDA requires the manufacturer to show the meter's accuracy as a percent (e.g., 94 percent accurate) on the box and corresponding test strips so that consumers can compare meters before purchasing. More expensive meters are not necessarily more accurate, although they often have features to make them easier to use. Individuals using standard glucose meters must keep a record of their blood glucose levels to share with their diabetes team. This can mean entering the time and numbers in a paper log or recording the information electronically by uploading it to a computer.

Test Strips

Test strips are specific to each brand of standard glucose meter; they are *not* interchangeable. Once a drop of blood has been drawn, it is applied to a test strip. The test strip is inserted into the meter, and the blood glucose level is shown on a screen. Each test strip can be used only once. The strips must be kept clean and dry and be used before their expiration date.

Because people with type 1 diabetes must check their blood glucose level frequently, test strips and lancets can become a substantial expense. According to a 2019 report by the *New York Times*, a box of 100 test strips can cost $100 without insurance. This has led to a thriving resale market, where people with insurance and small co-pays sell unused test strips at reduced rates to individuals who have no insurance coverage. Individuals buying test strips from resellers should make sure the box is unopened and that the strips have not expired.

Lancets

A lancet is a very small, sharp, narrow blade used to pierce the skin. Lancets come in different sizes, or gauges. The higher the gauge number, the thinner the lancet point. The lancet is placed in a spring-loaded plastic case called a lancet device. Clicking the button on the lancet device releases the spring and pushes the tip of the lancet through the skin to obtain a drop of blood for testing. For consistency and accuracy, blood is normally obtained from the tip of a finger. Some lancet devices come with lancets that are already loaded. The individual simply holds the device on the finger and clicks a button to release the lancet. Others require loading a new lancet each time the device is used. Some lancet devices allow the individual to set the depth of skin penetration.

Lancets come in sterile packaging and are intended to be used once and then discarded. Choosing the gauge of lancet and a lancet device depends on personal preference and cost. Experimentation will help the individual determine which combination of lancet and lancet device is easiest to use and causes the least painful finger stick.

Continuous Glucose Monitoring

CGMs consist of a sensor, a transmitter, and a receiver. They are more expensive than standard glucose meters. The sensor is a fine wire that is placed under the skin. It must be replaced every 5 to 14 days. Replacement can be done at home; it does not require a health care professional. The sensor measures the glucose level, not of blood, but of interstitial fluid, the fluid that exists between cells. Glucose in interstitial fluid generally reflects the glucose level in the blood, although if blood glucose levels rise or fall rapidly, there can be a lag time of 10–20 minutes before these changes are reflected in interstitial fluid. The sensor takes glucose readings every one to five minutes. In addition to a snapshot of blood glucose at one particular moment, CGMs can quickly show whether glucose levels are rising, falling, or remaining stable. This information can help head off hyper- or hypoglycemic episodes.

In a CGM, a transmitter sits on top of the sensor. This device looks like a large button. It sends information from the sensor wirelessly to a receiver. The receiver can be a separate device or an app on a smartphone. The receiver shows the current glucose reading and the direction the readings are trending. Some receivers will upload this information electronically to the cloud, where it can be shared with other individuals and the diabetes team. This feature allows parents to monitor their children's blood glucose levels when they are away from home. Transmitters are under development that send information to the individual's insulin pump (see "Insulin Delivery Systems" below) to alter the amount of insulin the pump releases.

Choosing a Glucose Meter

Choosing a glucose meter can be confusing. Every year, the magazine *Diabetes Forecast* compares both standard glucose meters and CGMs based on price of both the meter and test strips or replaceable sensors, accuracy, and special features. This comparison can help people with diabetes find the meter that best meets their needs. The following are some things to consider when choosing a meter:

• Cost. Cost of test strips and lancets or sensors should be included when figuring overall cost. The price of test strips can vary considerably.

• Insurance coverage. Insurance coverage is highly variable and can change yearly. Check what is covered before buying. Some insurance companies will only cover specific meters. Others will not cover CGM systems that have not been specifically approved for use in the age group of the user, even when prescribed by a doctor.

• Meter accuracy. This should be clearly listed on the box.

• Amount of dexterity needed to use the meter. Adults with arthritis or whose hands shake and children with small hands may have difficulty holding the meter and inserting the test strip.

• Special features. An extra-large screen, backlighting, or the ability to speak the results can assist individuals with impaired vision.

• Information storage and retrieval. Will the user have the skills to upload data into a computer and send it electronically to their diabetes team, or would the user prefer to manually record each reading? If so, will he or she record the information consistently?

• Privacy concerns. Some people are sensitive about revealing that they have diabetes and prefer standard glucose meters and manual recording of results to maintain privacy. With CGMs, it is more obvious that the individual has diabetes, and information that is shared electronically is more likely to be hacked or become public.

Ketone Testing

Ketones are compounds that build up in the blood and spill into the urine when the body breaks down fat for energy. They are a sign of hypoglycemia. People with type 1 diabetes should test their urine for ketones whenever their blood glucose level is 240 mg/dl (13.4 mmol/L) or higher. People with any type of diabetes should check for ketones in their urine when their blood glucose level is above 300 mg/dl (16.6 mmol/L) or when they are sick, stressed, pregnant, or have any signs of hypoglycemia.

Pregnant women with diabetes are often instructed to check for ketones every morning.

To test, the individual places a ketone test strip in the urine stream or a cup of collected urine. The strip will change color, indicating the level of ketones in the blood. If the tests show that small amounts of ketones are present, the test should be repeated in a few hours. Moderate or large amounts of ketones indicate that immediate action is necessary, and a doctor or diabetes educator should be contacted.

Insulin Delivery Systems

When insulin was first purified, the only way to administer it was by injection with a syringe and needle. Today, individuals have a choice of traditional syringe injection, injection with an insulin pen, or use of an implanted insulin pump. Some people may be able to use inhaled insulin, although this method is limited and is not popular. Each method has advantages and disadvantages.

Backup doses of insulin should always be available, regardless of the chosen delivery method. In the United States, if a person with diabetes is out of insulin and cannot reasonably reach a doctor for a prescription, any pharmacy, urgent care center, or hospital is required to make a supply of emergency insulin available without a prescription. This could happen if, for example, the delivery method fails (e.g., a pump stops working), the individual is seriously delayed while away from home, or in the event of a disaster—anything from a house fire to an earthquake. These facilities require the diabetic person to provide proof that he or she has diabetes. Usually showing an empty insulin vial, used insulin pen, or glucose meter is adequate proof. The insulin offered is usually intermediate acting NPH insulin and is intended to get the person through the immediate crisis only.

Syringe Injection

Inserting insulin into the body with a syringe and needle subcutaneously— that is, into the fatty layer under the skin but above the muscle—is the traditional way of injecting insulin. Most insulin sold in the United States is U-100, or 100 units of insulin per ml. Each vial of U-100 contains 10 ml of fluid, or 1,000 units of insulin. The accompanying syringe is marked in milliliters. Most types of insulin are clear, but NPH insulin is uniformly cloudy because of the way it is made, and it should be cloudy when used.

The diabetes team will demonstrate how to correctly draw a dose of insulin into the syringe and inject it. The injection site should be rotated to prevent damage to the fat under the skin. The preferred injection site is the abdomen between the ribs and the pelvis, excluding a 2-inch (5 cm) area surrounding the naval. Alternate injection sites are the back of the arm between the elbow and shoulder, and the top or outer edge of the of the thigh midway between the hip and knee. Most children can inject themselves by the age of nine, but they still need adult supervision to determine the correct dose and to draw it into the syringe.

Insulin to be injected by syringe must be kept away from heat or light. Unopened bottles should be stored in the refrigerator at between 36°F and 46°F (2.2°C and 7.7°C). Open bottles should be kept between 56°F and 80°F (13.3°C and 26.7°C). Insulin that is accidentally frozen should not be used, even if it thaws. Insulin exposed to high temperatures—for example, left in a hot car—should be discarded. Unless label instructions indicate otherwise, any insulin left in an opened bottle after 28 days should be discarded, except for bottles of NPH insulin, which can normally be used for 42 days after opening. All insulin has an expiration date and should not be used past that date.

Syringe injection is the least expensive way to take insulin. It also allows the individual to easily vary the dose or to mix two types of insulin—for example, rapid-acting and regular insulin—in the same dose. Disadvantages include the need to perform injections; the inconvenience of always keeping a vial of insulin, syringes, and a supply of sterile needles with one when away from home, and the potential for error in drawing the correct dose into the syringe.

Used syringes, needles, and lancets should not be tossed loose into the trash or recycled. The disposal of these items is regulated by individual states. The Safe Needle Disposal website (https://safeneedledisposal.org/) shows how to safely dispose of these items and lists disposal regulations by state and the locations of authorized disposal stations.

Insulin Pens

Insulin pens are an alternate way to inject insulin that many people find more convenient than syringe injection. They were introduced in 1985 by Novo Nordisk. In Europe, Asia, and Australia, about 95 percent of people who need insulin use insulin pens. They are less popular in the United States, partly because of uneven insurance coverage.

There are two types of pens: prefilled pens that are disposed of when empty and durable pens that can be refilled with a replaceable cartridge. Each cartridge contains 300 units of insulin. Both types of pens have a dial to adjust the amount of insulin to be injected and a way to see how many doses are left in the pen. Both types of pens require that a new injection needle be inserted at each use.

Insulin pens should be protected from extreme heat and freezing. Unopened pens should be kept in the refrigerator. Open pens can be kept at room temperature for 28 days or as indicated on the device instructions. The greatest advantage of insulin pens is convenience. Pens require less dexterity than using a vial and syringe, a benefit for children and the elderly. Studies have shown that dose accuracy of pens is consistently greater than with the vial-and-syringe method. Many people also find injection by pen both more discrete and less painful than using a syringe and needle. The greatest disadvantage is cost. In the United States, some insurance companies cover insulin pens, while others do not. Pens, which contain 3 ml of insulin (300 units) in 2018 cost between $98 and $300 without insurance. Another disadvantage of pens is that two types of insulin cannot be mixed in a pen.

Insulin Pumps

Insulin pumps are the newest type of insulin delivery system. These pumps normally use only rapid-acting insulin. The user can program the pump to provide a continuous flow of a small amount of insulin, with larger bolus doses before meals. There are two types of pumps: durable pumps and patch pumps. At the time this book was written, pump technology was evolving rapidly. Individuals interested in using an insulin pump should check with their diabetes educator about the latest features and advances that go beyond the general description below.

Durable pumps are about the size of a deck of cards and are made to last many years. They are worn outside the body on a belt around the waist or as an arm band. A durable pump consists of a programmable computer with display screen and an insulin delivery system. The computer controls a small motor that draws tiny amounts of insulin from an insulin reservoir in the pump. The correct amount of insulin must be programmed into the computer by the user.

The pump is connected by a plastic tube to an infusion set. The infusion set has a very small, thin plastic tube (less than 0.5 inches or 9 mm long) called a cannula that the user inserts subcutaneously using an insertion device to puncture the skin. The insertion site is usually in the abdomen. People who sweat a lot may need to hold the cannula in place with adhesive tape. Once the computer has been programmed and activated, the motor draws the correct amount of insulin into the tube. Insulin then flows through the tubing, into the cannula, and then into the body. Most pumps have a warning device to let the wearer know when blood glucose levels fall too low. Some will automatically stop the flow of insulin if glucose levels fall into the dangerously hypoglycemic range. Pumps can keep up to three months of information that can be downloaded to a computer to share with the diabetes team. This information is useful in spotting problems and trends. Insulin pumps are most often used with a continuous glucose monitor.

Most insulin pumps are used by people with type 1 diabetes and include a bolus dose calculator. The wearer puts his or her personal insulin-to-carbohydrate (I:C) ratio into the computer, along with a correction factor called the insulin sensitivity factor and the carbohydrate content of the meal. The computer then calculates approximately how much extra insulin (the bolus dose) is needed to cover the upcoming meal. Unlike the basal dose, which streams continuously, the bolus dose is given by pushing a button on the pump, usually about 15 minutes before each meal.

Unlike durable pumps, patch pumps are attached directly to the body. They have no tubing or infusion set. The computer, alarm mechanism, bolus calculator, and data storage are in a separate controller that communicates wirelessly with the patch pod. Before the pod is attached to the body, the user inserts insulin into a reservoir in the pod using a special needle. Patch reservoirs hold a minimum of 90 units and maximum of 200 units of insulin. The pod is then attached by an adhesive to the body. Once it is in place and the wireless connection is established, the pod injects the cannula automatically. Depending on the wearer's insulin usage, the pod can last 72 hours (the longest recommended usage time) or need to be changed more frequently. Once the pod is empty, it is discarded.

Advantages of insulin pumps are better blood glucose control and fewer incidents of hyper- or hypoglycemia. Many people find that they allow more flexibility in eating and exercising. Pumps avoid finger sticks. On the other hand, learning to correctly use an insulin pump requires extensive training and practice. The pump is only as good as the information programmed into it by the user.

Because pumps use only rapid-acting insulin, if the tubing, infusion set, or pod is dislodged, or if the insulin reservoir is empty, the individual will rapidly develop hypoglycemia that can easily progress to DKA. Accidents do happen, so it is essential that pump wearers have a backup supply of insulin; for example, an insulin pen, available at all times.

Another concern about insulin pumps arose in June 2019. A security flaw was detected in the software that controlled Medtronic's MiniMed 508 and MiniMed Paradigm insulin pumps. The United States Cybersecurity and Infrastructure Security Agency reported that the software flaw "may allow an attacker with adjacent access to one of the affected products to intercept, modify, or interfere with the wireless RF [radio frequency] communications to or from the product. This may allow attackers to read sensitive data, change pump settings, or control insulin delivery" (CISA 2019). The pumps were recalled and replaced with a version that did not use the flawed software.

A final disadvantage to insulin pump usage is cost. Insurance coverage is variable. Without insurance, the Academy of Managed Care Pharmacy estimated that in 2018, durable pumps cost between $4,500 and $6,500. With insurance, the co-pays ranged from $5 to $3,250. In addition, disposable supplies for these pumps cost about $1,500 per year without insurance and up to half that with insurance co-pays.

Inhaled Insulin

Inhaled insulin is rapid-acting insulin that can be used about 15 minutes before a meal by people with either type 1 or type 2 diabetes. People with type 1 diabetes must also use longer-acting insulin, which cannot be inhaled, for their basal dose. For some people with type 2 diabetes, inhaled insulin could be the only insulin they need, while others with insulin-dependent type 2 diabetes may need to supplement inhaled insulin with longer-acting, noninhaled insulin. Inhaled insulin comes in a cartridge in powdered form, with a single inhaled dose per cartridge.

The first inhaled insulin, Exurbera, was approved for use in the United States in 2006. It was a financial failure and was withdrawn from the market for financial reasons. Exurbera effectively lowered A1c, and, for some people with type 2 diabetes, completely eliminated the need to deliver insulin by injection. However, Exurbera could not be used by people who smoked and those who had recently quit smoking because smoking increased the risk of developing hypoglycemia. Its use increased respiratory infections and decreased lung function, and there was a slight but inconclusive indication that it was associated with an increase in lung cancer. In 2014, the FDA approved Afrezza, another inhaled insulin. It has the same benefits and drawbacks as Exurbera. Afrezza was still available in 2019 but was not widely used, and insurance coverage for the drug was inconsistent.

TYPE 2 DIABETES MANAGEMENT

Type 2 diabetes is not an autoimmune disease. The disorder develops because the body become resistant to insulin. Insulin resistance prohibits glucose from entering cells. Instead, glucose builds up in the blood, and hyperglycemia develops. Along with increasing insulin resistance, the amount of insulin the pancreas is able to make decreases. However, insulin-producing cells are not destroyed; they just do not function well enough to maintain health. Type 2 diabetes develops in people with certain risk factors, such as obesity; a sedentary lifestyle; a genetic tendency toward the disorder; and often, but not always, advanced age. (See chapter 3 for more on risk factors.)

As with type 1 diabetes, there is no cure for type 2 diabetes, but the disorder can be managed. Controlling blood glucose levels allows people to lead active and productive lives and reduces complications of the disorder. In addition, many people diagnosed with prediabetes are able to reverse this condition or prevent it from progressing to type 2 diabetes without using drugs, through diet and exercise. Prevention is discussed in chapter 8.

As with type 1 diabetes, the management goal of type 2 diabetes is maintaining blood glucose levels as close to normal as possible. However, since the factors that cause type 2 diabetes are different from those causing type 1, management strategies are also different. Type 2 can often be managed through careful attention to diet, exercise, and an appropriate drug regimen. Some people with type 2 diabetes, however, will eventually need insulin to remain healthy.

People with type 2 diabetes still need to check their blood glucose levels (see "Blood Glucose Monitoring" and "Glucose Meters," above), but usually they need to check much less often than people with type 1 diabetes. People newly diagnosed with type 2 diabetes may, however, temporarily need frequent testing to see how their bodies are responding to lifestyle changes and medication. People who are successful in managing their type 2 diabetes commit to seeing their doctor regularly, taking their medicine as prescribed, establishing an exercise routine, and monitoring their diets.

Lifestyle Management

The basic lifestyle management advice for people with prediabetes and diabetes can be summed up in four words: eat less; move more. For people who are overweight, as many people with type 2 diabetes are, losing weight is one of the most significant lifestyle changes they can make to manage the disorder. Any weight loss is good, but a loss of 10–15 percent of body weight can substantially lower blood glucose levels in almost every overweight person. A combination of controlled diet and regular exercise can lower glucose levels and reduce the need for medication.

Dietary Guidelines

The ADA does not recommend a specific "diabetes diet," believing that no single diet will meet the needs of every person with diabetes. Instead, they emphasize that meals should be based on a variety of healthy, nutrient-dense foods, be appealing to the individual, and be affordable. Portion control is equally important, as the overall dietary goal is to consume fewer calories. In addition, for best glucose control, meals should be eaten at regular intervals.

The ADA strongly encourages newly diagnosed individuals to work with registered dietitians or registered nutritionists to become educated about how different foods affect blood glucose, how to achieve portion control, the advantages of carbohydrate counting (see "Counting Carbohydrates" in "Type 1 Diabetes," above), and how to develop a healthy meal plan. A healthy meal plan should meet the diabetic individual's need for glucose control, be appealing enough to stay on for years, and be acceptable to the whole family. Some insurance plans will cover the cost of nutritionist or dietitian counselling.

Elements of a healthy diet appropriate for someone with type 2 diabetes and family members are outlined below. These are only general recommendations. More detailed information on healthy eating for people with diabetes can be found at the ADA website (http://www.diabetes.org) or at the website of the Academy of Nutrition and Dietetics (https://www.eatright.org). In addition, many cookbooks have been developed for people with diabetes; however, a dietitian or nutritionist is the best source of practical information for implementing these guidelines.

- Increase the amount of non-starchy vegetables, such as spinach, carrots, tomatoes, green beans, asparagus, peppers, summer squash, and turnips.

- Limit amounts of starchy vegetables, such as potatoes, corn, peas, acorn squash, and butternut squash by serving them less frequently and measuring servings.

- Choose whole grains over refined grains because whole grains are digested and absorbed more slowly, reducing the risk of glucose spiking after meals. For example, brown rice and whole-wheat flour are healthier choices than white rice and white flour. Whole grains also contain more nutrients. Quinoa, oats and oatmeal, whole barley, whole farro, and buckwheat are also good whole grain choices.

- Choose lean proteins, such as seafood, fish, and skinless chicken, and limit the amount of red meat. If eating red meat, choose cuts that are trimmed of visible fat. Pinto, kidney, navy, black, and similar beans, as well as meatless products that mimic meat products, such as vegetarian "chicken" nuggets and artificial meat "burgers" are good sources of low-fat protein.

- Reduce consumption of fats, especially saturated fats, which are fats from animal products, such as fatty meat, cheese, whole milk, and butter.

- Choose baked or steamed over fried foods because fats are especially high in calories and can raise cholesterol levels.
- Substitute fruits (if canned, packed in light syrup or fruit juice) for cookies, ice cream, candy, and similar foods that are high in sugar.
- Avoid regular soda, fruit drinks, energy drinks, sweet tea, and sweetened coffee. These drinks are high in sugar and rapidly raise blood glucose levels. Do drink plenty of water to stay hydrated. People with type 2 diabetes who drink alcoholic beverages should read the section on alcohol under "Type 1 Diabetes," above.

Exercise Guidelines

The exercise goal for people with type 2 diabetes is to sit less and move more. Exercise directly benefits a person with type 2 diabetes by lowering blood glucose levels. It causes muscles to use more glucose, thus decreasing the amount of glucose in the blood. Exercise also makes skeletal muscles more sensitive to insulin, lowering insulin resistance. Obesity is a risk factor for type 2 diabetes. The CDC estimates that 40 percent of Americans are obese. Exercise, combined with a healthy diet, helps people lose weight, which lowers blood glucose levels and reduces the risk of prediabetes progressing to type 2 diabetes and type 2 diabetes advancing to the point where the individual needs insulin to control blood glucose levels.

General exercise guidelines vary according to age. The American Academy of Pediatrics advises that children and teens with type 2 diabetes get 60 minutes of moderate to vigorous exercise daily and limit nonacademic screen time to a maximum of three hours per day. The exercise recommendation for adults ages 18–64 is 45 minutes of moderate exercise, such as brisk walking, five times per week. For Americans over the age of 65, the recommendation is 30 minutes of moderate exercise five times per week unless restricted by health or mobility. The ADA recommends a mixture of aerobic exercise and strength training as being most effective for people with type 2 diabetes. More information on exercising with type 2 diabetes can be found at the ADA website (http://www.diabetes.org).

Aerobic exercise lowers blood glucose levels, improves cardiovascular health, increases HDL (good) cholesterol, lowers LDL (bad) cholesterol, lowers blood pressure, improves sleep, boosts mood, and helps relieve stress. Low-impact aerobic exercises, such as water aerobics, can reduce chronic pain. Examples of aerobic exercise are brisk walking or jogging, swimming, water aerobics, bicycling, dancing, heavy cleaning, and gardening. The ADA recommends 30 minutes of aerobic exercise five times per week.

Strength training, also called resistance training, helps build muscle and keeps bones strong, reducing the risk of fracture when falling. Resistance exercises include weight lifting, working out with resistance bands, push-ups, sit-ups, and similar exercises. The ADA recommends strength training two or three times a week in addition to aerobic exercises.

Although studies show that people who join a structured exercise class or gym have better results than people who exercise alone, many people, especially in the over-65 age group, face barriers to structured programs. They may not have transportation to classes or cannot afford the cost of a gym membership. They may be overweight, have led sedentary lives for years, and feel uncomfortable exercising in front of other, more fit, people. In addition, many people in the over-65 age group have health problems, such as arthritis, that alter their ability to exercise.

The following suggestions may make it easier for people to get started and stick with an exercise program:

- Consult a doctor about appropriate exercises and any exercise limitations.
- Start slowly, with 10–15 minutes a day of exercise.
- Try not to let two days in a row pass without exercising.
- Consult a physical therapist, exercise physiologist, or personal trainer about exercises that provide the most benefit within the limitations of health and mobility restrictions.
- Add spontaneous exercise during the day. Increase steps walked by parking farther from stores. Stand up and do stretches or other exercises whenever commercials come on the television. At home, use canned food as weights to improve strength.
- Use a fitness tracker app or pedometer to measure progress.

Drugs to Manage Type 2 Diabetes

When changes in diet and exercise are not enough to bring blood glucose levels within the normal range, these efforts must be supplemented with drug therapy. Unlike insulin, which is injected, most drugs for type 2 diabetes are taken by mouth. There are many drug options for treating type 2 diabetes. Some drugs enhance certain aspects of glucose regulation, such as insulin production and insulin sensitivity. Others block chemical actions that normally decrease or inactivate insulin, while still others slow the absorption of carbohydrates or increase the excretion of glucose.

Drugs are grouped into classes based on how they work. As of 2019, there were 11 classes of drugs, in addition to insulin, that could be used to treat type 2 diabetes. Within each class, there can be multiple drugs with varying effectiveness, side effects, and cost. Often, people must take drugs from two or more classes to control their blood glucose level, but not all diabetes drugs can be taken together. People prescribed any new drug should provide a complete list of all over-the-counter and prescription drugs, supplements (e.g., vitamins and minerals), and herbal remedies they are taking, so a physician or pharmacist can explain the limitations and interactions of these remedies and the new drug being prescribed.

A general explanation of how each class of drugs works is given below, with examples of drugs in each class. New drugs to treat diabetes are being introduced as this book is being written in 2019. Many of the drugs mentioned have not been tested on children or pregnant and breast-feeding women. Before starting a drug, up-to-date information on both older and newly approved drugs should be obtained from a physician, pharmacist, or certified diabetes educator.

Note that in the sections below, the generic drug name is given first, with examples of the same drug sold under an American brand name in parentheses. People who travel outside their home countries should be familiar with the generic name of the drugs they take, as these remain the same across countries, while brand names for the same drug are often different. An additional consideration when filling prescriptions is that a generic drug is chemically equivalent to its corresponding brand name drug, but it is almost always less expensive.

Biguanides

Metformin (Glucophage, Fortamet, Glumetza, Riomet) is the only type 2 diabetes drug in this class. Developed in 1959 but only approved in the United States in 1990, metformin is recommended as the first-choice drug for treating type 2 diabetes by the American College of Physicians. It is also sometimes prescribed for people with prediabetes. Metformin decreases the amount of glycogen that is broken down into glucose by the liver by decreasing the amount of glucose absorbed from the intestine and by increasing sensitivity of cells to insulin, which allows more glucose to enter cells. This helps lower overall blood glucose levels, reduces A1c, and helps control rapid rises in blood glucose (glucose spiking) after meals. In some people, it promotes moderate weight loss.

Metformin is usually taken twice a day. It is safe, effective, and causes minimal side effects, the most common being nausea and diarrhea. It may reduce kidney function and is not appropriate for people whose kidney function is impaired. Metformin can be taken alone or in combination with sulfonylureas, thiazolidinediones, or some other diabetes drugs. It is often combined for convenience in a single pill with these other drugs and marketed under a separate brand name. As a generic, it is a relatively inexpensive diabetes drug.

Sulfonylureas

Three diabetes drugs are classified as sulfonylureas: glimepiride (Amaryl), glipizide (Glucotrol), and glyburide (Micronase, DiaBeta, Glynase PresTab). The first generation of these drugs was introduced in the 1950s. They were some of the first drugs used to treat type 2 diabetes. More effective sulfonylureas, with fewer side effects, became available in the 1980s.

Sulfonylureas work by stimulating beta cells of the pancreas to produce more insulin after meals. They are most effective in individuals who still retain moderate beta cell function. Glimepiride, introduced in 1995, lowers blood glucose levels and reduces A1c values, but it is also thought to reduce the amount of glycogen that is broken down into glucose by the liver and to decrease insulin resistance in cells. Sulfonylureas are often taken twice a day. The most common side effect is hypoglycemia. These drugs also may cause weight gain. The generic versions of these drugs are relatively inexpensive.

Meglitinide Derivatives

The diabetic meglitinides repaglinide (Prandin) and nateglinide (Starlix) have actions that are similar to sulfonylureas in stimulating insulin production, but they act much faster. Repaglinide was approved by the FDA in 1997, and nateglinide in 2000. Meglitinides are usually taken three times a day before meals and remain active for about four hours. The advantages of these drugs are that they are much less likely to cause hypoglycemia than sulfonylureas, and they are safe for people who are allergic to sulfonylureas. Disadvantages include the fact that they must be taken three times daily and can cause weight gain, nausea, and headaches. They are substantially more expensive than sulfonylureas.

Thiazolidinediones

Thiazolidinediones (TZDs) are also called glitazones. The TZDs pioglitazone (Actos) and rosiglitazone (Avandia) lower blood glucose levels by making skeletal muscle more sensitive to insulin so that muscle cells take up more glucose from the blood. They do not stimulate the pancreas to make more insulin. These drugs must be taken for 12 to 16 weeks to achieve maximal effect. They are often taken with diabetes drugs from other classes.

TZDs have several side effects that limit their use. They cause fluid retention and, thus, are poor choices for people with congestive heart failure or other fluid-retention issues, including macular edema, an eye disorder that can cause blindness. Also, their long-term use (one year or more) is associated with an increased risk of bone fracture, especially in women. Their use for two or more years appears to be associated with a slight increase in bladder cancer.

Alpha-glucosidase Inhibitors

Acarbose (Precose) and miglitol (Glyset) were approved by the FDA in the mid-1990s. They are taken before meals to slow the absorption of carbohydrates from the small intestine. This helps reduce glucose spiking after meals, but it does not change the total amount of carbohydrates that are absorbed. Their effect on A1c is modest, and their use is limited because they cause increased gas, stomach pain, and diarrhea.

Glucagon-Like Peptide-1 Agonists

Agonists are chemicals that stimulate an action. Their opposites are antagonists, which block an action. Incretins are agonist hormones made in the small intestine and colon that stimulate the release of insulin in response to eating food. They were discovered through the observation that, in a healthy person, the same amount of glucose given by mouth will cause a greater release of insulin from the pancreas than an equal amount of glucose given by injection. This led researchers to look for something in the digestive tract that signaled the pancreas to produce more insulin in a way that did not happen if glucose was injected directly into the bloodstream. This signal turned out to be several incretin hormones, the most important of which for treating type 2 diabetes, is glucagon-like peptide-1 (GLP-1). GLP-1 not only causes the release of insulin in response to food but also slows stomach emptying and reduces glucose spiking.

Glucagon-like peptide-1 (GLP-1) agonists are drugs that activate the same cells in the pancreas as naturally produced GLP-1. Like GLP-1, they stimulate the release of insulin only in the presence of food in the digestive tract, and they slow stomach emptying. GLI-1 agonists approved by the FDA as of 2019 are exenatide (Byetta, Bydureon), liraglutide (Victoza), dulaglutide (Trulicity), lixisenatide (Adlyxin), and semaglutide (Ozempic).

Most drugs used to manage type 2 diabetes are taken by mouth, but GLP-1 agonists are injected. Depending on the specific drug, they may be injected as often as twice daily or as infrequently as once a week. These drugs are not a first-line treatment for type 2 diabetes. They are used when blood glucose levels are poorly controlled with metformin, sulfonylureas, diet, and exercise. They reduce A1c levels and also reduce the chance of developing hypoglycemia when compared to sulfonylureas. In many people, they promote weight loss. Disadvantages include the need to inject these drugs and their cost. GLP-1 agonists are relatively new drugs. The first was approved by the FDA in 2014. The effects of long-term use are still being studied. These drugs are not appropriate for all individuals, especially those who have a family history of certain cancers.

Dipeptidyl-Peptidase 4 (DPP-4) Inhibitors

Dipeptidyl-peptidase 4 (DPP-4) inhibitors help slow the destruction of incretin hormones such as GLP-1, allowing them to stimulate the pancreas for a longer period. They are used most often when other drugs cannot provide good glucose control. This class of drugs includes sitagliptin (Januvia), saxagliptin (Onglyza), linagliptin (Tradjenta), and alogliptin (Nesina). These drugs are taken by mouth, usually once a day. They do not cause hypoglycemia, but they may increase respiratory infections, cause inflammation of the pancreas, and create unpleasant gastrointestinal symptoms. Some early research suggests that they may decrease the risk of bone fracture, but this finding has not been confirmed as of 2019.

Sodium-Glucose Cotransporter-2 (SGLT-2) Inhibitors

Drugs in this class, which includes canagliflozin (Invokana), dapagliflozin (Farxiga), empagliflozin (Jardiance), and ertugliflozin (Steglatro), block the reabsorption of glucose by the kidney. The glucose that is not reabsorbed is excreted in urine, thus lowering blood glucose levels. These drugs are most often taken in combination with other type 2 diabetes drugs. They can help with weight loss, but they also increase the risk of bladder and yeast infections, especially in women.

Bile Acid Sequestrants

Bile is a digestive fluid that is made in the liver and stored in the gallbladder, where it is released to aid in the absorption of fats and fat-soluble vitamins. Normally bile sequestrants are prescribed to lower cholesterol levels. One drug, colesevelam (Welchol), is also FDA approved as supplemental therapy in type 2 diabetes. It lowers LDL (bad) cholesterol in addition to blood glucose. How this drug works is not entirely clear. Its side effects are mainly gastrointestinal—nausea, gas, stomach pain, constipation, or diarrhea.

Dopamine-2 Agonists

Bromocriptine (Cycloset) is the only drug in this class that is FDA approved for the treatment of type 2 diabetes. Bromocriptine is taken once daily in the morning. It increases sensitivity of cells to glucose and reduces glucose spiking after meals. Its mechanism of action is unclear, although it appears to work in the hypothalamus, a part of the brain. The hypothalamus is located at the base of the brain and serves as a critical link between the nervous and endocrine systems. Its main function is to maintain homeostasis in the body.

Amylin Agonists

Amylin is a hormone secreted by pancreatic beta cells that reduces the production of glucagon, the hormone that stimulates conversion of glycogen in the liver into glucose and that slows stomach emptying. People with type 1 diabetes make no amylin because their beta cells are destroyed. People with type 2 diabetes have beta cells that function at a reduced level and. therefore, make less than optimal amounts of amylin. Pramlintide (Symlin) is the only amylin agonist approved by the FDA. It can be used by people with both type 1 and type 2 diabetes. Pramlintide is a synthetic version of amylin and mimics its actions. It is given as a subcutaneous injection using a prefilled pen before each meal. Individuals using pramlintide must check their blood glucose levels before eating and at bedtime, as the drug can cause hypoglycemia. Other side effects include nausea, vomiting, diarrhea, and dizziness. Pramlintide has substantial limitations on who can safely use it.

Insulin Use in Type 2 Diabetes

Type 2 diabetes is a progressive disorder. After many years, beta cell production of insulin may slow, and insulin resistance of cells may increase to the point where blood glucose levels can no longer be controlled with diet, exercise, and oral drugs. When this happens, a person with type 2 diabetes will need to inject insulin. This does not happen to everyone with type 2 diabetes, and it does not happen within a uniform time frame. The decision to start insulin must be made on an individual basis in consultation with the person's physician.

Insulin available to people with type 2 diabetes is the same as insulin used by people with type 1 diabetes and comes with the same need to check blood glucose levels frequently and to monitor carbohydrate consumption. Individuals who achieve the best control with insulin are those who are careful and conscientious about its use and who have a lifestyle that includes healthy meals at regular intervals. Anyone who is using or thinking about using insulin to manage type 2 diabetes should read the sections "All Insulin Is Not Alike," "Counting Carbohydrates," and "Blood Glucose Monitoring" under "Type 1 Diabetes," above.

Bariatric Surgery

Bariatric surgery, also known as metabolic surgery or weight loss surgery, is performed on the stomach and intestines for the purpose of weight loss. This surgery is not a cure for type 2 diabetes, but many obese people gain better control over their blood glucose level when they lose weight. For some people, blood glucose levels return to the normal range after this surgery. People who may be good candidates for bariatric surgery are those whose BMI is 35 or greater (see chapter 3 "Lifestyle and Environmental Risks" for more on BMI); have had difficulty achieving good blood glucose control with diet, exercise, and drugs; and are otherwise in good health.

There are several types of bariatric procedures. The one most commonly recommended for people with type 2 diabetes is gastric bypass surgery, also called Roux-en-Y surgery. This surgery significantly reduces the size of the stomach by stapling part of it shut. The new, smaller stomach pouch is then connected to the middle part of the small intestine. A smaller stomach pouch means that the individual feels full more quickly, and, by reducing the length of the small intestine, fewer nutrients are absorbed. Weight loss occurs, and often blood glucose levels drop.

This surgery is permanent, and, like all surgeries, carries significant risks and the potential for complications, as well as benefits. In addition, not all insurance companies cover this surgery for people with type 2 diabetes. Anyone considering bariatric surgery should research the procedure, discuss the risks and benefits with their physicians and get a second opinion before committing to the procedure.

GESTATIONAL DIABETES

Gestational diabetes is hyperglycemia that develops in a pregnant woman who did not have diabetes before she became pregnant. Special concerns in women who already have diabetes before they become pregnant are discussed in chapter 6. Women at high risk for gestational diabetes (see chapter 3 for risks) are screened early in pregnancy. Other women are screened around the beginning of the third trimester of pregnancy (see "Oral Glucose Tolerance Test," above).

During pregnancy, the placenta produces a hormone called human placental lactogen, also called human chorionic somatomammotropin. This hormone increases insulin resistance so that the woman's cells take in less glucose, and blood glucose rises. This is normal. The extra glucose in the blood provides nutrients that allow the baby to grow. A second hormone, placental growth hormone, is supposed to help regulate the mother's blood glucose level so that the developing baby gets all the nutrients it needs. However, in gestational diabetes, it appears that this regulation does not work well. Blood glucose levels rise and stay high, resulting in hyperglycemia in the mother and excess growth of the baby. This is why women with gestational diabetes often have babies weighing 10 pounds (4.5 kg) or more. Babies of mothers with gestational diabetes are three times more likely to be delivered by cesarean section and are four times more likely to spend time in a neonatal intensive care unit. Large babies delivered vaginally have an increased rate of birth injuries.

Many women with gestational diabetes can control their blood glucose levels through diet and exercise. Diet should be supervised by a registered dietitian or certified diabetes educator. Women are often told to eat multiple small meals each day, limit carbohydrates, and exercise a minimum of 30 minutes daily. When diet and exercise fail to control hyperglycemia, they may be prescribed insulin or the biguanide metformin and/or a sulfonylurea. Insulin may be preferred because it is definitely safe to use in pregnancy. Metformin and sulfonylureas cross the placenta. They do not appear to harm the developing baby, although long-term effects are still being studied.

6

Long-Term Prognosis and Potential Complications

A great deal of the medical care and expense of diabetes revolves around minimizing and managing complications that can decrease quality of life and shorten life span. Complications from diabetes can affect almost every part of the body from the brain to the feet and can be acute or chronic. Acute complications come on rapidly and can often be resolved in a relatively short time. Chronic complications usually arise slowly, last a long time, and are treatable but not often curable. Complications will be described in this chapter, while prevention and delay of complications will be discussed in chapter 8.

ACUTE COMPLICATIONS

Two acute complications, DKA and hypoglycemia, have already been discussed in chapter 5. A third acute complication, hyperosmolar hyperglycemic state (HHS), although rare, can occur in people with type 2 diabetes. HHS, also sometimes called hyperosmolar hyperglycemic nonketotic syndrome, is a condition in which all the electrolytes (chemicals) in the blood become too concentrated. When this occurs, water is drawn out of body cells and into blood vessels to help restore the correct concentration of chemicals.

The movement of water out of cells causes them to become seriously dehydrated.

In HHS, blood glucose levels soar as high as 900 mg/dl or 50 mmol/L (100 mg/dl or 5.6 mmol/dl is normal). This increase occurs without causing the production of ketones. That means that HHS happens only in people with type 2 diabetes. People with type 1 diabetes have ketones in their blood and will develop DKA when untreated blood glucose is extremely high. HHS almost always begins with an infection or a recent stressful event, such as a heart attack or surgery.

Normally, when blood glucose levels rise, a person feels thirsty and drinks more fluids to relieve thirst. This increases urine output and helps the kidneys get rid of excess glucose. However, in HHS, the individual does not drink enough and becomes progressively more dehydrated, to the point that glucose levels increase drastically, and blood chemistry is altered. This condition is especially common in the frail elderly who are mobility or communication impaired, have dementia, or have neurological conditions that interfere with their perceptions of thirst. These individuals are most often in nursing homes or in situations where there is no easy access to water on demand. Certain drugs frequently given to the elderly, such as steroids, diuretics, and anticonvulsants, can accelerate the rise in blood glucose.

The best way to prevent HHS is to make sure that diabetic individuals have easy and frequent access to fluids and that they drink adequate amounts. People with diabetes also need to have their blood glucose levels checked several times a day during illness or after stressful events. Increased checking can be a problem in the group most likely to develop HHS, but frequent blood glucose testing allows corrective action to be taken as soon as glucose levels begin to rise. HHS is a medical emergency, but it gives few visible warning signs, such as the nausea or vomiting that occur with DKA. Instead, blood pressure drops until the individual slips into a coma. Treatment of HHS involves insulin and replacement fluids to restore the chemical balance of the blood. Even with treatment, the death rate is about 40 percent.

CHRONIC COMPLICATIONS

Chronic complications are much more common among diabetics than are acute complications. They tend to progress slowly so that damage goes unnoticed until they cause a dramatic event, such as a stroke, or interfere with quality of life by causing decreased vision, slow wound healing, or nerve damage. These complications occur in people with both type 1 and type 2 diabetes but can also occur for reasons independent of diabetes.

Three types of factors affect the development of complications associated with diabetes. The first are factors that the individual cannot change. These include genetic inheritance, age, and gender. Some people, because of these uncontrollable factors, will be at increased risk of developing complications associated with diabetes.

The second set of factors affecting whether a person develops diabetic complications are issues that can be modified. These include smoking, obesity, physical inactivity, high cholesterol, high triglyceride levels, and hypertension (high blood pressure). Diet and lifestyle choices affect these factors. The degree to which they are controlled can change the likelihood that a person with diabetes will develop complications. People without diabetes can also develop health complications from these factors.

The third of these factors is the management of diabetes. Diabetes management is considered a partially modifiable factor in determining whether an individual will develop complications. Multiple long-term studies of people with type 1 or type 2 diabetes have shown that individuals who maintain blood glucose levels that are close to normal over a period of years are much less likely to develop life-altering complications.

CARDIOVASCULAR COMPLICATIONS

The cardiovascular system consists of the heart and all the blood vessels in the body. Blocked or severely narrowed blood vessels can cause heart attack, stroke, high blood pressure, and peripheral artery disease. Diabetes does not directly cause these events—they also occur in people without diabetes—but the rate at which they occur is much higher in people with either type 1 or type 2 diabetes. According to the American Heart Association, heart disease is the leading cause of death in people with diabetes. At least 68 percent of people over the age of 65 with diabetes die from some form of heart disease. In addition, diabetics develop heart disease at a younger age than nondiabetics.

Lifestyle factors, such as obesity, low physical activity, high cholesterol levels, high triglyceride levels, and smoking make both diabetic and nondiabetic individuals more vulnerable to heart disease. The more of these factors a person has, the higher the risk of developing atherosclerosis. Atherosclerosis occurs when fatty material made mainly of cholesterol is deposited on the wall of an artery. Over time, these deposits harden and are called plaque. Plaque narrows the diameter of the artery and reduces the amount of "give," or flexibility, in the artery wall. At this point, the condition becomes a more severe disorder called arteriosclerosis, or, more commonly, hardening of the arteries. Arteriosclerosis develops slowly over a long time and gives few warning signs until the condition is severe.

Although an individual cannot change the effects of age, gender, and genetic inheritance on the development of arteriosclerosis, minimizing the lifestyle factors mentioned above can prevent or slow its development. For diabetics, however, high blood glucose is an additional risk factor that cannot be eliminated through lifestyle changes, although it may be moderated through a combination of diet and drug treatment.

Researchers are just beginning to understand why high blood glucose is a risk factor for heart disease. Arteries are large blood vessels that carry blood away from the heart, while veins carry blood back to the heart. Arteries have thicker, more muscular walls than veins because they must withstand increased pressure each time the heart contracts and pushes blood into them for distribution around the body. As of 2019, researchers have determined that high glucose levels cause arteries to contract more strongly than normal, which means that they narrow more than the blood vessels of a person with normal glucose levels. Preliminary research studies suggest that this increased contraction and narrowing is linked to the presence of one or more regulatory proteins that are higher in people with diabetes.

The health significance of narrowed arteries is that the heart must work harder to push blood through the body. This increased pressure is reflected in higher blood pressure readings. In addition, narrowed arteries are more likely to become blocked. If preliminary research findings are verified, they could explain why people with diabetes are at higher risk for developing heart disease.

Coronary Artery Disease

Two main coronary arteries and their branches supply the heart with oxygen. When these arteries narrow, blood flow to the heart is reduced, a sign of coronary artery disease (CAD). At first, CAD produces no symptoms. When a coronary artery is about 70 percent blocked, the individual may experience angina. Angina feels like pressure and pain in the chest. Pain may spread to the left arm, neck, jaw, or shoulder. It develops most often when a person is active and disappears if one rests. Sometimes the individual also feels sweaty and short of breath. Not everyone with CAD experiences angina. This is especially true of diabetics, because diabetes also causes nerve damage that may interfere with the perception of pain (see "Nervous System Complications" later in this chapter).

A heart attack, formally called a myocardial infarction, occurs when one of the coronary arteries is blocked to the degree that the heart is deprived of oxygen. This results in damage to the heart muscle. The most obvious symptoms of a heart attack are intense pain and pressure below the breastbone that can spread to the arm, neck, or jaw. Other symptoms include heavy sweating, nausea, severe indigestion, shortness of breath, weakness, dizziness, or fainting. On the other hand, some people, especially people with diabetes, experience only mild or no symptoms. Any suggestion that an individual is having a heart attack requires *immediate* medical attention because half of all people who die from heart attacks do so within the first hour after symptoms begin.

Stroke

There are two types of strokes. Hemorrhagic strokes occur when a blood vessel in the brain weakens and bleeds. Ischemic strokes occur when blood flow to the brain is blocked. Eighty-seven percent of strokes are ischemic strokes, which are the focus of this section. As with CAD, the risk of stroke is affected by nonmodifiable factors, lifestyle factors, and diabetes. An individual with either type 1 or type 2 diabetes is two to four times more likely to have a stroke than a nondiabetic person; 16 percent of diabetics die from stroke.

Strokes occur because blood clots tend to develop at the places where plaque has formed on artery walls. Over time, these blood clots can grow to block the artery, or they can break off and travel though the circulatory system until they come to a blood vessel that is too narrow for them to pass through. In either case, when the artery leads to or is within the brain, a stroke occurs, and the portion of the brain deprived of oxygen is damaged.

Strokes come on rapidly. Warning signs include sudden weakness or numbness of the face, arm, or leg on one side of the body. Sudden change in vision, trouble talking or understanding speech, and sudden severe headache can also indicate a stroke. Often dizziness, unsteadiness, or a fall occur along with these symptoms. Sometimes these symptoms appear and then disappear within 10–15 minutes. This is typical of a transient ischemic attack (TIA), sometimes called a mini stroke or warning stroke. TIAs occur when blockage of blood flow to the brain is temporary. TIAs should be treated as medical emergencies because when symptoms begin, it is not possible to know their severity. After a TIA, medication may help prevent recurrence or a more severe stroke. As with CAD, people with diabetes, on average, experience strokes at a younger age than nondiabetics.

Peripheral Arterial Disease

Peripheral arteries are arteries in the arms, hands, legs, and feet. They deliver blood to areas outside the chest and abdomen. Peripheral arterial disease (PAD) is related to the development of arteriosclerosis. In diabetics with PAD, fatty deposits and hardened plaque usually form in the arteries below the knee. Narrowed arteries and reduced blood flow then cause lower leg pain and cramps, a condition called claudication. Pain is often associated with exercise and may disappear after resting. PAD also can cause numbness, tingling, cold lower legs and feet, and wounds that are slow to heal (see "Foot Complications" later in this chapter).

PAD has the same risk factors as CAD. Like other cardiovascular complications, PAD occurs earlier in people who have diabetes than those who do not. It is especially common in diabetics who smoke, often developing in these people in their fifties. PAD increases the risk of gangrene and lower limb amputation. Exercise may prevent early PAD from progressing. More advanced PAD can be treated with drugs or sometimes with vascular surgery.

EYE COMPLICATIONS

Diabetes can damage many different parts of the eye, including the lens, vitreous humor, and retina. It causes a variety of conditions, ranging from pain to blurred vision to blindness. Different complications result from damage to different parts of the eye. Figure 6.1 illustrates the basic anatomy of the eye.

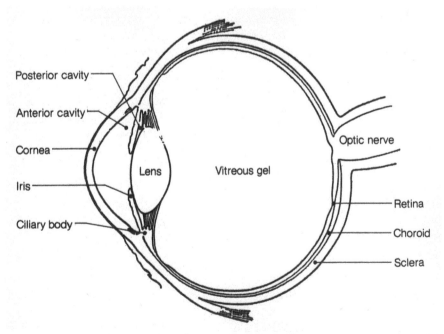

Figure 6.1   Diagram of the Eye (National Eye Institute, https://nei.nih.gov/health /eyediagram)

Clear tissue, called the cornea, covers the exterior of the eye. It protects against germs and foreign material, such as dust. The cornea contains no blood vessels. It is nourished by fluid that fills a space behind the cornea, called the anterior cavity. The iris and the lens are located in the anterior cavity. The iris is the colored part of the eye. It consists of a ring of muscular tissue that surrounds the pupil, or dark part of the eye. By contracting or relaxing, the iris controls the size of the pupil, which determines the amount of light entering the eye.

The lens is transparent flexible tissue located behind the iris and pupil. Tiny muscles can change the shape of the lens. The ability of the lens to change shape allows a person to switch seamlessly from seeing a nearby object to one that is far away. Together, the cornea and the lens focus light on the retina on the back, interior wall of the eye. A clear, jelly-like substance called the vitreous humor fills the space between the lens and the retina.

The retina is made up of millions of specialized nerve cells, called rods and cones, that line the back of the eye. The center of the retina is called the macula. The macula contains mainly cones and is responsible for distinguishing fine details and seeing colors. The area surrounding the macula contains mainly rods. It is responsible for peripheral vision and vision in low light. Both rods and cones convert light into nerve impulses that are transmitted by the optic nerve at the back of the retina to the brain, where they are converted into the image that we see.

Diabetic Retinopathy

Retinopathy is a general term for damage to the retina. Diabetic retinopathy is the principal eye complication associated with diabetes. It is the leading cause of new blindness diagnoses in Americans under the age of 60. The development of this disorder is related to the length of time the individual has had diabetes and the degree to which blood glucose is maintained at close to normal levels. About 28 percent of diabetics aged 40 years and older have some degree of retinopathy.

Individuals with type 1, type 2, and even gestational diabetes can develop diabetic retinopathy. The first five years after diagnosis, people with type 1 diabetes show no signs of the disorder, but after 10 to 15 years, one-quarter to one-half have some retinal damage. After 15 years, 75 percent or more of type 1 diabetics have significant symptoms. At 30 years after diagnosis, close to 100 percent of people with type 1 diabetes have significant diabetic retinopathy, and many have become blind.

In people with type 2 diabetes, the development of diabetic retinopathy depends on the length of time they have had diabetes. About 23 percent of people with type 2 diabetes develop retinopathy after 13 years, 41 percent after 16 years, and 60 percent after having diabetes for more than 16 years. This compares to less than 15 percent of the population that is not diabetic. Pregnant women with gestational diabetes have a 10 percent chance of developing diabetic retinopathy.

Although researchers have not pinpointed the exact cause of diabetic retinopathy, multiple factors appear to be involved. One is increased clumping of blood cells, commonly seen in people with diabetes. Excess clumping tends to reduce blood flow and block capillaries (tiny blood vessels) in the retina. This deprives retinal cells of oxygen and nutrients. Another factor is that in people with diabetes, some excess glucose is converted to other types of carbohydrates, such as sorbitol and dulcitol, that appear to make retinal capillaries weaken, bulge, and leak.

Regardless of the causes, diabetic retinopathy goes through several stages, beginning as nonproliferative retinopathy and progressing to serious proliferative retinopathy and blindness.

Nonproliferative retinopathy begins with small bulges in retinal capillaries. These bulges are called microaneurysms. They can be seen during an ophthalmic examination, but diabetic individuals initially experience no change in their vision. At this point, the disorder is considered mild.

As it progresses to moderate and severe nonproliferative retinopathy, more microaneurysms appear. Some microaneurysms break and bleed. Capillaries begin to leak, allowing proteins to escape the circulatory system and settle in the retina. Other capillaries become blocked, depriving the retinal cells of oxygen. Gradually, these conditions spread throughout the retina. Over time, the individual may see floaters (black spots in the field of vision), develop blurry or distorted vision, and experience progressive vision loss.

As cells of the retina are gradually deprived of a normal blood supply, they begin secreting a growth factor that stimulates the development of new blood vessels. Once new blood vessels begin to grow, the condition is known as proliferative diabetic retinopathy. Instead of replacing blood vessels that are damaged, the new blood vessels grow on the interior surface of the retina and into the vitreous humor. This interferes with the reception of light by cells in the retina. The new blood vessels are fragile and prone to leaking and breaking. Scar tissue forms that can pull rod and cone cells of the retina away from the back wall of the eye, a condition called retinal detachment. Once detached, these cells die, and vision is permanently lost.

Diabetic Macular Edema

Diabetic macular edema (DME) is the accumulation of fluid in the macula, or center of the retina. The macula is involved in discriminating among fine details, such as printed letters or facial features, and in distinguishing colors. People with DME develop blurry, distorted vision and may perceive colors as less vivid than normal. The condition develops because damaged blood vessels leak fluid that accumulates in the retina. DME is an extremely common cause of blindness in diabetic individuals.

About 750,000 Americans out of the 7.7 million who have diabetic retinopathy will develop DME. It is most common among African Americans, most likely because this group has the highest rate of diabetes and because among African Americans, diabetes and its complications often go undiagnosed for a long time due to barriers in accessing health care.

DME can happen at any stage of diabetic retinopathy, although it is most common in the later, more severe stages. People with poorly controlled type 2 diabetes are at highest risk. High blood pressure aggravates the condition. Macular edema has other causes that are independent of diabetes, including damage from eye infections, eye surgery, and age-related macular degeneration.

Glaucoma and Diabetes

Glaucoma develops when pressure increases in the eye as the result of fluid buildup in the anterior chamber. Excess pressure causes irreversible damage to the optic nerve and results in vision loss and blindness. Type 2 diabetes, along with genetic inheritance, use of steroid eye drops, eye injury, and eye infections, are risk factors for developing glaucoma. People with type 2 diabetes are twice as likely to develop glaucoma as people who do not have diabetes.

Open-angle glaucoma is the most common form of the disorder and is the type of glaucoma most people with diabetes develop, although it also has other causes. Medication delivered as eye drops or pills is usually prescribed to help control pressure buildup and prevent vision loss. Early detection is essential to preserving vision because once vision is lost due to excess pressure in the eye, it cannot be restored.

Neovascular glaucoma is a rare type of glaucoma that is always associated with diabetes. It develops in people with proliferative diabetic retinopathy when new blood vessels grow into the iris and block the normal drainage of fluid from the anterior chamber of the eye. It is much more difficult to treat than open-angle glaucoma. Laser or traditional surgery to allow fluid to drain may be needed.

Diabetic Cataracts

Cataracts develop when the clear lens of the eye becomes cloudy. They are common in individuals over 60 years of age and have other causes besides diabetes. In people with diabetes, cataracts tend to develop earlier, often in individuals in their thirties and forties. Over time, cloudiness causes impaired vision. Left untreated, blindness can result.

People with either type 1 or type 2 diabetes are susceptible to developing diabetic cataracts, especially if their blood glucose level is poorly controlled. These cataracts are sometimes called sugar cataracts. The reason sugar cataracts develop is not completely clear. They are thought to be related to the conversion of excess glucose into the carbohydrate sorbitol, as mentioned above in the discussion of diabetic retinopathy. Accumulation of sorbitol in the lens alters the fluid balance of lens tissue and causes it to break down. As the lens fibers degenerate, the lens becomes opaque, resulting in impaired vision. Cataracts can be treated with outpatient surgery, but people with diabetes are more likely to have post-surgery complications, such as the acceleration of diabetic retinopathy, macular edema, eye inflammation, and poorer vision compared to individuals without diabetes.

NERVOUS SYSTEM COMPLICATIONS

Diabetic neuropathy is nerve damage caused by diabetes. In people with type 1 diabetes, the damage tends to occur after many years. In people with type 2 diabetes, nerve impairment is seen much sooner after a diagnosis and generally occurs earlier in men than in women. About half of all Americans with diabetes have some degree of diabetic neuropathy. Rates are similar in the United Kingdom.

The underlying cause of diabetic nerve damage is not known, but the greatest risk factor is a long period of high blood glucose. Other factors that increase the likelihood of developing diabetic neuropathy include high cholesterol, high triglycerides, high blood pressure, obesity, smoking, and heavy alcohol use. Symptoms develop gradually, and many people are not aware of the condition until nerve damage has already occurred; about 7.5 percent of diabetics already have some degree of neuropathy by the time they are diagnosed with diabetes.

Diabetic neuropathy can be diagnosed through symptoms and blood tests for diabetes. Nerve conduction tests that indicate the health of nerve fibers may also be done. A simple light touch on the sole of the foot—a common place for early nerve damage—will indicate whether feeling in the foot has been lost. Many people who have diabetic neuropathy also have diabetic retinopathy and should be evaluated by an ophthalmologist as soon as diabetic neuropathy is diagnosed.

Diabetic neuropathy can be staged to indicate its severity. The stages are as follows:

- N0: No neuropathy
- N1a: The individual does not feel any symptoms, but signs of neuropathy can be detected by certain blood and nerve conduction tests.
- N2a: Symptoms are mild. Individuals are able to walk in the normal heel-to-toe fashion, where the heel hits the ground first. This is known as heel walking.
- N2b: Symptoms are severe. Individuals can no longer heel walk.
- N3: Disabling neuropathy. Use of a wheelchair is usually necessary.

Peripheral Diabetic Neuropathy

Peripheral diabetic neuropathy is the most common of the four types of diabetic neuropathy. Peripheral indicates that these symptoms occur in nerves that are far from the center of the body, in the arms, hands, legs, and feet. Usually the feet and legs are affected first. Initially, pain is more common at night. Both sides of the body tend to be affected at about the same time. Damage frequently occurs before the individual notices any symptoms.

The earliest symptoms include cold feet and hands, numbness, a tingling or burning sensation in the affected body part, and reduced ability to feel pain. More advanced symptoms include sharp cramps and pains, especially in the legs; extreme sensitivity to touch; muscle weakness in the hands and feet; loss of balance; and increased foot problems, such as deformed toes (hammer toe), joint pain, foot ulcers, and slow wound healing (see "Foot Complications" later in this chapter). Diabetic neuropathy cannot be cured, although good glucose control, physical therapy, and drugs to manage pain can help control symptoms.

Proximal Neuropathy

Proximal neuropathy, also called diabetic amyotrophy or radiculoplexus neuropathy, is the second most common type of diabetic neuropathy. It affects the muscles of the thigh, buttocks, and hips and causes them to weaken. This type of diabetic neuropathy is more common in people with type 2 diabetes and the elderly. Sometimes the disorder causes a sharp pain down the leg (sciatica). People with proximal neuropathy also have trouble rising from a sitting position.

Symptoms of proximal neuropathy come on suddenly and can be severe. Treatment involves pain medication and physical therapy. Symptoms may get worse before they get better, although they generally improve over time with treatment.

Autonomic Neuropathy

The autonomic nervous system generally controls involuntary actions. Some autonomic functions include the regulation of body temperature, heart rate, digestion, blood pressure, and sexual arousal. When the nerves controlling these functions are damaged by diabetes, the following symptoms can occur: problems controlling body temperature, with increased or decreased sweating; dizziness; a sharp drop in blood pressure when going from sitting to standing (orthostatic hypotension); trouble swallowing; and slow stomach emptying that causes bloating and nausea.

Loss of appetite makes it difficult for the individual to recognize hypoglycemia. Other symptoms of autonomic neuropathy include constipation, diarrhea, or a mix of both; urinary tract infections, poor bladder emptying and loss of bladder control; visual difficulty in adjusting to changing degrees of light; and erectile dysfunction (ED) (men) and vaginal dryness (women). Some people with diabetes fail to recognize that they are having a heart attack because the nerves to the heart are damaged, and the sensation of pain is reduced. Treatment is symptom specific.

Focal Neuropathy

The three neuropathies described above are polyneuropathies, meaning they affect multiple nerves. However, focal neuropathy, also called mononeuropathy, is damage to a single nerve. Pain can develop suddenly in the foot, shin, front of the thigh, chest, or arm. It can also develop in nerves of the neck and eye, causing partial facial paralysis, double vision, or eye pain.

This disorder occurs most frequently in older adults. For example, between 15 and 20 percent of people with diabetes have carpal tunnel syndrome, which, among other causes, may result from focal neuropathy.

Researchers believe that high blood glucose levels damage the nerve in the wrist that passes through the carpal tunnel and controls sensation and movement in the thumb and first three fingers of the hand. Some British studies suggest that developing carpal tunnel syndrome is a predictor for developing diabetes, although there are also other causes for carpal tunnel syndrome. Of the four types of diabetic neuropathies, symptoms of focal neuropathies are the ones that are most likely to go away without treatment, but they may take weeks to months to resolve.

FOOT COMPLICATIONS

Feet are often underappreciated parts of the body, but they are truly amazing mechanical constructions, consisting of 23 bones; 33 joints; and over 100 muscles, tendons, and ligaments. In other words, there is a lot in the foot that can go wrong. Foot problems can develop in anyone, but they are much more common in people with diabetes and have more profound effects on health than in nondiabetic individuals.

Foot problems are worsened by several diabetic complications, discussed earlier in this chapter. Diabetic peripheral neuropathy, for example, can cause loss of feeling in the feet. As a result, minor injuries, such as blisters, small cuts, or painless ulcers often go unnoticed until the foot becomes infected. In addition, as arteriosclerosis and peripheral artery disease develop, blood flow to the feet is impaired. Capillaries become blocked or weakened. If they break down, the body may fail to repair them.

When blood flow is reduced, cells receive less oxygen and nutrients. The skin becomes shiny, thin, and easily damaged. More importantly, wound healing is slowed. The immune system is already depressed in people with diabetes because high glucose levels tend to cause immune system cells to clump. Combined with poor circulation and lack of feeling, ulcers can form that allow bacteria to penetrate deep into the foot. In the worst cases, toes, feet, or legs must be amputated to prevent infection that would otherwise spread throughout the body, causing death.

Structural Complications

Diabetic individuals are susceptible to structural changes in the foot that can interfere with balance and mobility. Hammertoes are toes that curl at one or both joints at the end of the toe. The development of hammertoe has a genetic component (they run in families independently of diabetes), but hammertoe is also caused by muscle weakness that develops with diabetic neuropathy. Curling of the toe(s) alters the way a person walks, causing more pressure on the ball of the foot, where calluses often develop. The tops of the toes also rub against the shoe and become red and sore as skin is worn away.

Hammertoe is usually accommodated with special shoes that provide more room in the toe box or that are made of soft material that is less irritating to bent toes. Severe hammertoe can be treated with surgery, but given the complex structure of the foot, the surgery can cause other complications.

Charcot's foot is the most serious foot deformity associated with diabetes. It is caused by joint dislocations and bone fractures that gradually result in the destruction of bone and soft tissue. This eventually makes walking impossible. Although uncommon in the general population, as many as 2.5 percent of people with diabetes develop this disorder; however, of these, fewer than 10 percent develop the disorder in both feet.

Some studies have found that Charcot's foot is three times more common in men than women. Most people who develop Charcot's foot are older than the age of 50; have had diabetes for more than 10 years; and have other symptoms, such as loss of feeling in their feet and diabetic eye and kidney complications.

Foot Infections

Anyone can develop a foot infection, but people with diabetes not only have more of them, they also have a more difficult time curing their infections than nondiabetics. Because of this vulnerability, people with diabetes need to check their feet daily to identify any foot problems early. Foot problems that are ignored can develop into serious conditions that affect quality of life.

Athlete's foot (*Tinea pedis*), is a common fungal infection that causes itching and cracking of the skin, usually between the toes. For healthy people, treatment with an over-the-counter antifungal cream usually cures athlete's foot. People with diabetes, however, may need to take oral prescription medication to clear the infection. The concern with athlete's foot in diabetics, as with other foot infections, is that bacteria can enter the foot through the cracked skin and penetrate deep into the soft tissue. Bacteria are not killed by antifungal medication, and deep foot infections can result.

The risk of fungal infections under the toenails is three times greater in people with diabetes than in nondiabetics. The nails become thick and dark yellow or brown. Eventually, they may crumble. Curing fungal nail infections usually requires taking prescription pills. In severe cases, in addition to drug treatment, a doctor may need to surgically remove the nail and infected tissue.

Foot ulcers are open sores that can develop any time the skin is broken, such as when a blister breaks; a person steps on something sharp; or when thin, fragile, or dry skin cracks or is worn away. Untrimmed calluses can also break down into foot ulcers. These ulcers commonly develop on the ball of the foot or under the big toe. About 15 percent of people with diabetes will develop a diabetic foot ulcer. Diabetes prevents foot ulcers from healing at a normal rate. This is especially true in people with poorly controlled blood glucose levels.

Foot ulcers are often overlooked or ignored because they are usually painless. Nevertheless, they are one of the most potentially serious complications of diabetes because they allow tissues and bones of the foot to become infected. In recent years, a small but increasing number of foot ulcers in diabetics have become infected with antibiotic-resistant bacteria, creating a potentially fatal health hazard. A health care provider should see all foot ulcers as soon as they are discovered. Left untreated, they can develop into any of the following conditions, listed below, in order of severity:

- abscesses or locally infected spots, characterized by pockets of pus
- cellulitis, in which infection spreads to the fat underlying the skin
- osteomyelitis, an infection of the bones of the foot that can result in structural changes, such as Charcot's foot
- Gangrene, where tissue dies, becomes black and smelly, and rots as a result of the combination of infection and poor circulation. Treating gangrene can require amputation of toes, foot, or lower leg. Between 14 and 24 percent of people with diabetes who develop an ulcer will end up having an amputation. This amounts to about 230 amputations every day in the United States due to diabetes.

SKIN COMPLICATIONS

Infections can occur on the skin in other parts of the body besides the feet. Like foot infections in diabetics, they are often slow to respond to treatment. Any skin rashes should be brought to the attention of a health care provider. Self-treatment is not recommended. Fungal infections are treated either with over-the-counter or prescription antifungal sprays, creams, or occasionally prescription pills. Keeping the susceptible area dry and maintaining good blood glucose control can reduce recurrence.

Although anyone can acquire a fungal infection, some infections are more common in people with diabetes. *Candida albicans* is a yeast that grows in moist areas of the body. When it grows in the mouth, it appears as a white curd-like growth. It looks the same when it grows in the vagina, and it is very itchy. When found where skin rubs against skin, such as in the groin or under the breast or arms, it forms an itchy red rash.

Tinea cruris causes the fungal infection commonly known as jock itch. Symptoms include an itching, burning, red, scaly, ring-shaped rash with raised edges that appears on the inner thigh, groin, and around the anus. Women can develop jock itch, but it is more common in men.

Ringworm is closely related to jock itch and athlete's foot (*Tinea pedis*). Ringworm can infect any part of the body (*Tinea corporis*) or the scalp (*Tinea capitis*). It forms circular red rashes with raised edges. Untreated, these circular rashes can merge to form blisters.

Bacterial skin infections are also more common in people with diabetes. Some infect only the outer layer of the skin, while more serious infections invade the deeper layers of the skin. Small surface infections can usually be treated with antibacterial creams. More extensive surface infections and infections of deeper layers often require oral antibiotics and, in severe cases, intravenous antibiotics. Like fungal infections, bacterial infections do not go away on their own. They should be brought to the attention of a health care provider as soon as they are noticed.

Some of the more common or more serious bacterial skin infections that affect diabetic individuals, especially in those over the age of 50, are listed below:

- Impetigo is a surface skin infection caused by staphylococcus or streptococcus bacteria. It begins with a red pimple that fills with pus, breaks open, and then crusts over. In rare cases, the underlying tissue can become infected, causing cellulitis, which is a much more serious infection.

- Erythrasma is an infection of the surface layer of the skin caused by the bacterium *Corynebacterium minutissimum*. Initially it forms a pink or red rash that fades to scaly, brownish, itchy patches. It is found most often in moist areas where skin rubs against skin, particularly under the arms, under the breasts, and in the genital area. A variant of erythrasma can also infect the feet and cause painless fissures between the toes, particularly in people with type 2 diabetes.

- Cellulitis is a serious infection that is usually caused by staphylococcal or streptococcal bacteria that infect the deeper layers of the skin. The skin becomes warm, red, tender, and swollen. The individual may have a fever and feel ill. Although cellulitis can develop in any part of the body, it rarely occurs in both legs simultaneously. Left untreated, bacteria can move into the bloodstream and cause very serious illness. Cellulitis is usually treated with oral antibiotics but, if advanced, may require hospitalization and intravenous antibiotics. Cellulitis is not contagious.

- Erysipelas is an infection of the second, deeper layer of skin. The skin becomes red, hot, shiny, and swollen. The individual may feel ill with fever or chills. Most cases occur either on the face or the legs. Erysipelas is caused by streptococcus bacteria. Severe cases may require use of intravenous antibiotics to prevent cellulitis from developing.

- Necrotizing fasciitis, commonly known as flesh-eating disease, is an uncommon but life-threatening infection that kills the fascia, which is deep tissue that covers muscle. Soon the muscle becomes infected and dies. Over half the cases involve more than one type of bacteria, and antibiotic-resistant bacteria are involved in about one-third of cases. People with poor blood circulation, especially to the legs and feet, are more likely to develop necrotizing fasciitis. Symptoms include severe pain and red, warm, skin with blisters. Gangrene often develops. This requires immediate removal of the dead tissue and possibly amputation.

KIDNEY COMPLICATIONS

Diabetic kidney disease (DKD), also known as diabetic nephropathy, is the leading cause of kidney disease in the United States. An estimated 25 percent of Americans with diabetes will develop the disease. However, the prevalence of DKD is not evenly distributed. It is between three and six times more common among African Americans, Mexican Americans, and Native Americans. The rate is especially high among members of the Pima tribe of Arizona, where by the age of 20, half of all individuals with diabetes will have developed DKD.

The kidneys are fist-sized organs, weighing about 5 ounces (140 g) and located on either side and toward the back of the upper abdomen. They help maintain the fluid and chemical balance of the body by filtering blood at the rate of about 1 quart (1 L) per minute and removing excess fluid, chemicals such as salt, and waste products. These leave the body as urine. Although almost everyone is born with two kidneys, one is sufficient to carry out this function.

Each kidney is composed of about one million nephrons. Blood is filtered and cleaned as it passes through a cluster of capillaries in the nephron. Blood cells and large molecules remain in the capillaries, while water and small molecules pass across the capillary walls and into a tubule. Needed fluid and chemicals are reabsorbed into the circulatory system from the tubules. Excess fluid and waste products remain in the tubules and are collected in the bladder before leaving the body as urine.

As with many complications of diabetes (e.g., diabetic retinopathy, PAD, and wound healing), sustained high blood glucose levels damage the capillaries in the nephron. Once the capillaries are weakened, blood cannot be properly filtered or cleansed, and DKD develops. A protein called albumin that should be reabsorbed begins to be excreted in urine. Measuring the amount of albumin in urine gives an indication of the degree of damage and the stage of DKD.

Kidney disease is assessed in stages. Initially, the individual may show no symptoms, even though damage to the nephrons has occurred. As the disease progresses, the individual generally feels unwell, may have an irregular heartbeat; nausea and vomiting; and, most commonly, water retention (edema) in the legs and feet. The final stage of DKD is known as end-stage renal disease (ESRD). At this point, both kidneys are damaged to the degree that life can be maintained only by a kidney transplant or dialysis (artificial cleansing of the blood, typically three times per week).

Most people with type 1 diabetes show some changes in kidney function after having diabetes for five years. Between 30 and 40 percent progress to serious kidney disease over the next 25 years. Of those with serious disease, between 20 and 40 percent progress to ESRD.

The longer people have type 2 diabetes, the more likely they are to develop DKD. About 3 percent of people with type 2 diabetes already have kidney damage at the time they are diagnosed with diabetes. About 10–20 percent with type 2 diabetes ultimately progress to ESRD. Consistently high blood glucose levels, high blood pressure, smoking, obesity, and genetic inheritance all increase the risk of developing serious DKD.

GASTROINTESTINAL COMPLICATIONS

The speed at which food moves through the gastrointestinal system affects how rapidly nutrients are absorbed into the blood. When nerves that trigger movement of food through the gastrointestinal system are damaged by high blood glucose levels or inhibited by medication, a mismatch between glucose in the blood and available insulin can develop. This creates periods of hypo- and hyperglycemia and difficulty in bowel control. The longer people have had diabetes, the more likely they are to develop some of the gastrointestinal complications listed below.

Gastroparesis

Gastroparesis is delayed stomach emptying in the absence of physical obstruction. The delay often causes nausea, vomiting, abdominal pain, and a feeling of fullness after eating only a small amount of food. Although gastroparesis can have other causes, it is a common complication of diabetes. Estimates suggest that between 27 and 65 percent of people with type 1 diabetes and up to 30 percent of people with type 2 diabetes have some degree of gastroparesis. The disorder is more common in women than in men.

The cause of gastroparesis in diabetics appears to be damage from high blood glucose to nerves that stimulate stomach emptying. Certain diabetes drugs, such as metformin, also slow stomach emptying and can worsen the problem. Delayed stomach emptying can result in wide swings in blood glucose because the absorption of nutrients does not match the available insulin. This is especially true in people with type 1 diabetes who inject rapid-acting insulin. Recommended treatment is to eat smaller, more frequent meals; avoid difficult to digest foods; take medication to treat nausea; and, when possible, avoid drugs that slow stomach emptying.

Diabetic Enteropathy

Diabetic enteropathy is a fancy way of saying difficulty in bowel control caused by diabetes. It can involve diarrhea; constipation; or, often, a combination of the two. The cause appears to be damage to the nerves that stimulate movement of food through the intestines. Changes in gut bacteria from high blood glucose levels may also be a factor. Treatment aims to relieve symptoms and normalize bowel movements.

Some diabetes medications increase the likelihood of developing diarrhea. This occurs to an estimated 10 percent of people taking metformin and 20 percent of people taking alpha-glucosidase inhibitors (e.g., Precose and Glyset). Dipeptidyl-peptidase 4 (DPP-4) inhibitors (e.g., Januvia, Onglyza, Tradjenta, Nesina) may also increase bowel problems. See chapter 5 for more on these drugs.

People with long-standing diabetes may also experience fecal incontinence. This occurs when nerves around the anus are damaged, and muscle tone is lost. Consequently, the individual cannot always control bowel movements. Leaks of feces occur most often at night. This can create social and psychological stress (see "Psychological Complications" later in this chapter).

Gastroesophageal Reflux Disease

Gastroesophageal Reflux Disease, better known as heartburn, is more common in people with diabetes than in nondiabetic individuals. Obesity is also a contributing factor in developing heartburn. A circular muscle (the lower esophageal sphincter) is located where the esophagus meets the stomach. It is designed to close when food is in the stomach. If the muscle does not close tightly, a slurry of stomach secretions and partially digested food can backflow into the lower end of the esophagus. This mixture is very acidic and can cause a burning feeling in the throat and chest. Over time, it will damage cells of the esophagus, potentially causing inflammation, scar tissue formation, and changes in esophageal cells, a condition known as Barrett's esophagus. Barrett's esophagus increases the risk of developing esophageal cancer. Recommended treatment is to eat smaller meals, avoid acidic foods and alcohol, and take medication that reduces the production of stomach acid.

LIVER COMPLICATIONS

Nonalcoholic fatty liver disease (NAFLD) is the excess accumulation of fat in the liver not related to alcohol consumption. It describes two conditions, fatty liver and nonalcoholic steatohepatitis. NAFLD is associated with obesity and insulin resistance in type 2 diabetes. It is the most common liver disease in the United States. Most people with diabetes have fatty liver. They rarely experience symptoms, but their blood tests may show elevated liver enzymes.

If damage to the liver occurs along with fat accumulation, the disorder is called nonalcoholic steatohepatitis or NASH. NASH can cause liver inflammation and can progress to the formation of fibrous tissue and irreversible liver scarring that are the hallmarks of cirrhosis, a serious liver disease. NASH symptoms may include fatigue, weakness, and a dull ache in the upper right part of the abdomen. Both forms of fatty liver disease can also be caused by excessive alcohol consumption, unrelated to diabetes.

ORAL COMPLICATIONS

According to the American Dental Association, 20 percent of teeth that are lost are linked to diabetes. The most common dental complication is periodontal disease. The first signs of periodontal disease are red, swollen gums that bleed easily. This condition is called gingivitis. It can be controlled by good dental hygiene, including daily brushing, flossing, and regular cleanings by a dental hygienist. Left untreated, gingivitis can progress to periodontitis, a much more serious infection. In periodontitis, infection causes the gums to pull away from the teeth. The teeth can then loosen and fall out. The infected gums also cause persistent bad breath. Treatment involves special deep cleaning of the infected area by a dentist; medication; and, in severe cases, gum surgery.

Diabetes can also increase the chance of the fungus *Candida albicans* growing in the mouth, where it is commonly called thrush. The fungus forms white, curd-like growths on the gums, cheeks, and tongue. These patches can turn into open sores that are slow to heal. Treatment involves prescription medicine and, if the individual wears dentures, soaking them daily in a prescription solution to kill fungi.

Diabetes-caused damage to the nerves that stimulate the production of saliva can result in permanent dry mouth, a condition medically called xerostomia. Not only is dry mouth uncomfortable, the lack of saliva makes it easier for cavities to develop. Treatment involves prescription medicine, increased attention to dental hygiene to prevent the development of cavities, and not smoking.

SEXUAL COMPLICATIONS

Diabetes can affect the sex life of both men and women on two levels: physical and psychological. Often, these are intertwined, with diminished physical performance and sexual enjoyment leading to depression, shame, and negative self-image. There are many reasons for sexual dysfunction besides diabetes, but when diabetes is the cause or a contributing factor, it is usually because high blood glucose has damaged nerves and blood vessels that are involved in sexual response. In addition, both men and women can experience hypoglycemia during or just after sex, just as they can from any unplanned exercise.

Male Sexual Complications

Men's sexual complications from diabetes are more easily recognized and better documented than complications women experience. The most common complication is ED—the inability to achieve and maintain an erection. Men with diabetes are three times more likely to develop ED than nondiabetic men, and they develop it at a younger age, sometimes as early as their thirties. Eventually, about half of all diabetic men will develop ED.

The American Diabetes Association (ADA) estimates that between 10 and 20 percent of cases of diabetic ED are caused by stress, depression, low self-esteem, and fear of sexual failure instead of physical complications (see "Psychological Complications," below). Diabetic men with ED also tend to have lower than normal testosterone levels. A blood test can determine testosterone levels. ED can sometimes be treated with prescription drugs, counselling, and a change in the individual's diabetic care plan. Damage to nerves in the penis cannot be repaired. This damage can also cause delayed or impaired ejaculation.

Penile curvature, also called Peyronie's disease, is also more common in men with diabetes than in nondiabetic men. Scar tissue causes the penis to curve when erect, making sexual intercourse uncomfortable or difficult. In diabetic men, Peyronie's diseases is associated with ED, obesity, and smoking.

Diabetes can affect male fertility through ED and low testosterone. In addition, some studies have found that men with high blood glucose levels have an increased number of changes in the DNA of their sperm that may reduce sperm motility and fertility. This has been found in both men with prediabetes and men with poorly controlled diabetes. Obesity was a contributing factor in both groups of men.

Female Sexual Complications

Women's sexual complications from diabetes are less visible than men's. They include lack of sexual desire, the inability to be or stay aroused, painful intercourse caused by vaginal dryness, reduced feeling in the genitals, and the inability to achieve orgasm. Vaginal dryness often develops from nerve damage to the tissue that secretes vaginal lubricants. Nerve damage from high blood glucose also causes diminished sensation. Women with diabetes are also likely to have more frequent vaginal yeast infections and more bladder infections because high blood glucose levels encourage fungal and bacterial growth. Women's sexual response, like that of men, is affected by depression, low-self, esteem, and fear of failure.

Blood glucose levels in premenopausal women are affected by the hormones that regulate the menstrual cycle, creating another complication. Some hormones make the body more resistant to insulin at certain times in the ovulatory cycle. For example, it is common for blood glucose levels to rise for three to five days around the time of menstruation and then gradually return to normal.

The interaction between hormones and insulin may also affect a woman's choice of birth control methods. Some women find the hormones in birth control pills make it more difficult to regulate their blood glucose. Also, some thiazolidinediones (e.g., Actos, Avandia) used to treat type 2 diabetes (see chapter 5) make the body less responsive to the estrogen. For women taking low-dose birth control pills and these diabetes drugs, breakthrough bleeding or an unplanned pregnancy can occur. Women should discuss their birth control concerns with both their gynecologists and their diabetic educators in order to choose the most appropriate form of contraception for their situation.

Obesity, high blood pressure, insulin resistance, and diabetes are strongly correlated with a condition called polycystic ovary syndrome (PCOS). PCOS is a hormonal imbalance that causes irregular menstrual cycles and the formation of fluid-filled cysts (sacs) in the ovaries that disrupt ovulation. It is a common cause of infertility in women. Although diabetes is not a direct cause of PCOS, it is often a reason why women with type 2 diabetes have difficulty becoming pregnant.

PSYCHOLOGICAL COMPLICATIONS

A diabetes diagnosis is a life-changing event. The diagnosis triggers changes in diet, exercise, and the daily routine. It places extra responsibility on the individual to monitor blood glucose and take medication in the proper amount and at the proper time. It can cause worry about complications; stress over the financial burden of the disorder; and anxiety about how these changes may be accepted by family, friends, and employers. Over time, most people with diabetes go through periods of denial, frustration, fear, and burnout. The disorder also affects their families and friends (see chapter 7).

According to the Centers for Disease Control and Prevention, people with either type 1 or type 2 diabetes are two to three times more likely than nondiabetics to develop clinical depression. Of these, only between one-quarter and one-half receive the proper diagnosis and treatment. People with diabetes, especially women, are also at increased risk for anxiety and eating disorders. In women with type 1 diabetes, bulimia is the most common eating disorder. Women with type 2 diabetes are more likely to become binge eaters.

Diabetes Distress

Diabetes distress is a collection of negative emotions that include depression, anxiety, stress, frustration, and feelings of burnout. Because these feelings do not rise to the level of a mental health disorder, they are often overlooked and left untreated, even though they are very common. In addition, wide swings in blood glucose levels can cause fluctuations in mood, leaving the diabetic feeling both guilty for failure to regulate blood glucose and emotionally out of control. It is estimated that within any 18-month period, between one-third and one-half of all people with diabetes will experience an episode of diabetes distress. Caregivers, especially parents of children with type 1 diabetes, can experience similar feelings of distress (see chapter 7).

Doctors at the University of California, San Francisco have developed a screening test to diagnose diabetes distress in people with type 2 diabetes. A screen for people with type 1 diabetes is under development. The type 2 test looks at four areas of concerns that place an additional burden on the psychological well-being of diabetics. These are:

•   management issues, such as distress related to diet, exercise, and taking medications;

•   worry about complications;

•   concerns about quality of care; and

•   stress from social aspects of the disorder.

Once recognized, symptoms of diabetes distress can be treated with individual and family therapy, stress reduction techniques, and support groups.

COMPLICATIONS OF PREGNANCY

Pregnancy creates a whole new set of complications for women with diabetes. Some women who did not have diabetes before becoming pregnant will develop gestational diabetes during pregnancy. Others who already have type 1 or type 2 diabetes will need to modify their diabetes care programs and comply with them closely to protect their health and the health of the developing fetuses.

Gestational Diabetes Complications

Gestational diabetes is a form of diabetes that develops in some women when they become pregnant. During pregnancy, the placenta, which connects the developing fetus to the mother's blood supply, produces hormones that create insulin resistance in cells. If the woman does not make enough insulin to counteract this, blood glucose levels rise, and diabetes develops. Gestational diabetes normally does not occur until after the twentieth week of pregnancy, and usually much later. It is most common among African American, Latina, and Native American women. Obesity and a family history of gestational diabetes are also risk factors.

Complications from gestational diabetes can occur in both mother and baby. Women with gestational diabetes are more likely to develop pre-eclampsia. The first sign of preeclampsia is high blood pressure (multiple readings of 140/90 mm Hg or higher). Another early sign is protein in the urine, which indicates kidney stress. Other signs include nausea, vomiting, severe headaches, vision changes, and decreased urine volume. Preeclampsia is a serious condition that, if left untreated, can lead to eclampsia, which involves potentially life-threatening seizures.

Some women with gestational diabetes can control their blood glucose levels through changes in diet and exercise. Others require bed rest and insulin injections or oral diabetes medications.

High blood glucose levels also cause the fetus to grow larger than normal, a condition called macrosomia. This may necessitate birth by cesarean section or cause injury to the baby or mother during a vaginal birth. Although gestational diabetes normally goes away after the baby is born, the mother has as much as a 60 percent chance of developing type 2 diabetes within 10 years of giving birth. This risk can be reduced to 25 percent if the woman maintains a healthy weight, eats a healthy diet, and exercises. Women who have had gestational diabetes with one pregnancy are likely to develop it again during subsequent pregnancies.

Gestational diabetes can cause complications for the baby as well as the mother. The disorder may cause early labor. Babies born early sometimes have difficulty breathing, a condition called respiratory distress syndrome. Even when the baby is not born early, respiratory distress syndrome can occur in babies born to mothers with gestational diabetes. These babies can also experience hypoglycemia and seizures shortly after birth. The pancreas of a baby whose mother has gestational diabetes usually has been making extra insulin to compensate for the mother's high blood glucose levels. After the baby leaves the womb and is no longer exposed to the mother's blood, this extra insulin can cause a period of hypoglycemia.

Later in life, babies born to mothers with gestational diabetes are more likely to develop type 2 diabetes. However, because gestational diabetes does not develop until near the end of the second trimester, these babies have the same risk of miscarriage and birth defects as babies born to nondiabetic mothers.

Pregnancy Complications with Established Diabetes

Special concerns exist when women already have type 1 or type 2 diabetes before becoming pregnant. The degree of complication depends on how long the woman has had diabetes, how well controlled her blood glucose levels are, and whether she already has blood vessel or kidney complications. In ideal circumstances, women will have their blood glucose levels as close to normal as possible *before* they try to conceive. This is important because most of the baby's major organs are formed by seven weeks after the last menstrual period, when many women do not realize that they are pregnant, and fetal organ formation is affected by high blood glucose levels.

Poorly controlled glucose levels during the first trimester increase the risk of birth defects in the fetus. In nondiabetic women and in diabetic women whose blood glucose is well controlled and close to normal, the rate of fetuses with a major birth defect ranges from 1 to 4 percent. In women with type 1 diabetes and poorly controlled blood glucose, the rate of major birth defects is between 5 and 10 percent. In addition, these women have a 15 to 20 percent chance of miscarriage.

All women with diabetes need to monitor their blood glucose levels more frequently while they are pregnant. Diabetic care plans will adjust throughout the pregnancy. Women with type 1 diabetes will likely need to increase their insulin injections, but this can be tricky and can sometimes result in hypoglycemia and ketoacidosis. Women with type 2 diabetes will likely need to change their medications, as many drugs used to treat type 2 diabetes are not safe to take during pregnancy. These women may need to switch to insulin injections, depending on the extent of their diabetes.

Insulin needs of women change rapidly after birth, gradually returning to more stable prepregnancy levels. Women who breastfeed will require additional ongoing adjustments in their diabetic care plans. Care from a doctor and diabetes educator experienced in helping women through pregnancy will help minimize complications for both mother and baby.

LONG-TERM PROGNOSIS

In both type 1 and type 2 diabetes, tight control of blood glucose levels leads to fewer complications and a longer life. The significance of maintaining near-normal blood glucose levels cannot be underestimated.

On average, people with type 1 diabetes live about 11 years less than non-diabetics. However, this statistic can be misleading. About 60 percent of people with type 1 diabetes do not develop serious complications, but the remainder develop life-limiting and fatal complications. The risk of an early death is greatest among people who develop type 1 diabetes before the age of 15, and, in this group, the risk of early death to men is twice that of women. Most people with type 1 diabetes die from heart and kidney complications.

For people with type 2 diabetes, the overall death rate of is twice that of people of the same age who are not diabetic. Individual life expectancy depends on maintaining blood glucose levels as near normal as possible, as well as the length of time the individual has had diabetes. Kidney and heart complications are most likely to be fatal. For example, coronary heart disease occurs two to four times more often in people with diabetes than those without the disorder.

7

Effects on Family and Friends

Diabetes management affects more than the person with the diagnosis. The people affected and the extent to which the disorder impacts their daily lives depends on whether the friend or family member has type 1 or type 2 diabetes. Because type 1 is usually diagnosed in children, it places a greater demand on family and caregivers. People with type 2 diabetes are more likely to be able to manage their own medication, unless they are elderly or incapacitated.

All diabetics tend to be concerned that other people's perceptions of their diagnosis will affect their work and social lives. The International Diabetes Foundation and the United Nations declared the family and diabetes as the theme for World Diabetes Day in 2018 and 2019.

Because type 1 and type 2 diabetes affect family and friends in different ways, they are discussed separately.

EFFECTS OF TYPE 1 DIABETES

Every year, about 18,000 children under 19 years old are newly diagnosed with type 1 diabetes in the United States. This diagnosis is a life-changing event for the child and the child's family. The learning curve is steep, the time commitment great, and the responsibility a heavy and unexpected burden. Beyond the family, childhood diabetes affects the child's caregivers, teachers, coaches, parents of the child's friends, and anyone else who interacts regularly with the child. The responsibility changes over time as the child matures, and parents must balance their child's need for more independence against his or her ability and willingness to comply with insulin administration and diet.

Effects on Parents

Having a child receive a diagnosis of type 1 diabetes is a shock. After the numbness wears off, parents experience a range of emotions. These tend to resurface as the child matures, and challenges of managing the disorder change. The first emotion parents often experience is denial that their child has diabetes or that it is a lifelong disorder. They may also deny that their lives will change in significant ways. Some parents become angry that doctors cannot cure the disorder. Others ask, "Why me? What did I do to deserve this?" These are normal reactions.

Research has shown that a child's type 1 diagnosis causes both immediate and long-term stress for parents. In one small study (38 families), about one-fourth of the parents met the American Psychological Association criteria for post-traumatic stress disorder (PTSD) six weeks after their child received a type 1 diagnosis. Half of the remaining parents had some symptoms of PTSD, but not enough for a formal diagnosis. A significant number still showed some symptoms of PTSD after one year. Another study found that up to one-third of parental stress was associated with whether parents believed they could handle the child's diabetes, the level of involvement in the child's daily care, and fear of hypoglycemic episodes. These stresses often added to the normal stresses of daily life (e.g., financial, job, or marital stress). As a result, parents of children with type 1 diabetes were more likely to experience depression and anxiety. In some cases, high parental stress increased stress in the diabetic child and interfered with the ability of the parent to learn how to manage their child's disorder. This resulted in poor blood glucose control in the child.

Guilt often accompanies a child's diagnosis. Parents may feel that they should have recognized that their child had a serious disorder and done something about it sooner. This is especially true when the child has been diagnosed after a life-threatening bout of DKA. Other parents look for an explanation in something they have done or failed to do that caused the disorder. They may not understand or accept that there is nothing they could have done to change or prevent the diagnosis (see chapter 8). Type 1 diabetes is an autoimmune disorder. Although the exact cause is unknown, it is likely to be a combination of genetic factors and an unidentified environmental trigger (see chapter 3), both of which are beyond parental control.

The Learning Curve

Once a child has been diagnosed with type 1 diabetes, the education process begins. Learning about the way insulin works, how to check blood glucose levels and give injections, counting carbohydrates, and recognizing when a child is experiencing hypoglycemia can feel like a crushing responsibility. On a practical level, parents must adjust their priorities. This can be especially difficult for single-parent families and families where both parents work full time. Who will take the child to frequent medical appointments? Who will be responsible for checking the child's blood glucose levels up to 10 times each day? Who will give the insulin shots? Will the whole family need to change their diet? What do school and daycare personnel need to know to keep the child safe? Can they meet the child's need for insulin and a regulated diet? What should a parent say to the newly diagnosed child and his or her siblings and relatives about the disorder?

The logistics of coping with a new diabetes diagnoses inevitably cause anxiety and frustration within the family. In addition, fear of doing something wrong that may harm the child—miscalculating an insulin dose or failing to recognize signs of hypoglycemia—often increase anxiety. Parental frustration, anger, and depression are common. Although these feelings decrease slightly after the first year, depression and anxiety tend to reappear as the child becomes a teenager and strives for more independence.

While parents are learning to cope with their emotions, the diabetic child is coping with his or her own feelings. The emotions the child expresses and the way he or she handles them affect the entire family. Depending on their age and understanding of the disorder, children can cycle through multiple emotions, including denial, depression, anxiety, guilt, fear of death or health consequences, excessive dependence on parents, fear of being different, embarrassment, isolation, anger, frustration, resentment, and defiance.

Parents and teens often experience a particularly difficult time. Teens are old enough to check their own blood glucose levels and give their own injections. Some use insulin pumps and continuous glucose monitoring systems that give them more flexibility in managing the disorder but that also adds a new level of responsibility. Even with an insulin pump, there are still restrictions.

Teens want to be like their peers—eat what their peers eat, play sports, go on overnight trips, date, and drive. They may be embarrassed by the steps needed to manage their diabetes in a way that allows them to participate in these activities. While parents worry about long-term complications of high blood glucose (see chapter 6), their children are normal teens, focused on today and not potential complications in 10 or 20 years. Adolescent rebellion against the diabetes management plan is common, accompanied by a period of poor glycemic control and a higher risk of hypoglycemic episodes. This can be especially dangerous if the teen experiments with alcohol or drugs. Diabetes distress and burnout, discussed in chapter 6, are common in both parents and teens.

Effects on Siblings

Whatever happens to one member of the family affects all members, so it is not surprising that if a child is diagnosed with type 1 diabetes, his or her siblings are also affected. The ability of siblings to adjust to the new diagnosis varies with their age, maturity, and the parents' and the type 1 child's response to the diagnosis. Some studies have found that younger siblings find it harder to adjust, but older siblings are more sensitive to the changes taking place in the family. Younger children may act out, while older siblings may suppress their feelings as a way of coping. Siblings of the same gender as the diagnosed child tend to have more difficulty coping than opposite gender siblings. The ability of siblings to cope with the changes a type 1 diagnosis brings varies from family to family. Nevertheless, adjustment in siblings of all ages and genders tends to improve over time.

The first emotion many siblings feel is fear. A child newly diagnosed with type 1 diabetes has often had a serious hypoglycemic episode and needs to be hospitalized for several days until he or she can be stabilized and the parents' education begun. Other children in the family may fear that their brother or sister will die. The family routine is disrupted. The parents may stay at the hospital with the ill child, while the other children are left with caregivers. Depending on their age and experience, siblings may have no idea what diabetes is and can be afraid that they also will "catch" it.

Over time, siblings experience many of the same feelings as their parents—anger, guilt, fear, resentment, frustration, anxiety, and depression. Newly diagnosed children may need to have their blood glucose levels checked up to 10 times a day and have insulin injections up to five times a day. Younger siblings may be afraid of the testing and injection materials. Older siblings may resent the attention given the diabetic child. Teens may be expected to help with monitoring and injections and be afraid of or resent the added responsibility. They also may feel embarrassed about explaining their sibling's disorder to friends.

Food is a common source of contention. A parent's decision to stop buying sugary and high-carbohydrate foods and fill the house with foods the diabetic child can eat may become a source of resentment for nondiabetic siblings. Not only does the food served at meals change, the entire process surrounding mealtimes—checking blood glucose levels, counting carbohydrates, injecting insulin—is anything but restful. In addition, meals must be eaten at certain times for the best glycemic control, limiting dining flexibility. Some families choose to continue purchasing foods that are high in sugar and carbohydrates for nondiabetic siblings. The diabetic child may resent that he or she cannot eat them or be tempted to cheat on the diabetic management plan and sneak a treat.

All children react to stress their parents feel. Studies show that the better parents adapt to the diabetes management plan, the more easily siblings adjust, and the better the glycemic control is of the diabetic child. After adjusting to the new routine, some families note that the effects of having a diabetic child are not all negative. They say everyone eats healthier meals and, in some instances, they have become closer as a family.

No matter how well adjusted they are, every family needs a break from diabetes management to prevent burnout. The American Diabetes Association (ADA) sponsors day, overnight, and family camps for diabetic children as young as four and as old as 17. These camps allow kids to be with others like themselves where they do not have to explain their disorder. At the same time, parents and siblings get a break from the daily routine of diabetes management. Financial aid is often available to allow children from all income levels to attend these camps.

EDUCATING OTHERS

Families with a diabetic child do not live in a vacuum. The child must still go to school, make friends, participate in extracurricular activities, and travel. For the safety of the child and the peace of mind of the parents, adults the child spends time with need to be educated about diabetes, warning signs of hypoglycemia, and how to respond in an emergency.

Diabetes at School

Accommodations at school for a child with type 1 diabetes vary according to the age of the child, the diabetes management plan, federal and state law, and school district policy. Under federal law, diabetes is considered a disability. The federal Americans with Disabilities Act of 1990 prohibits discrimination against people with disabilities. It applies to daycare centers, preschools, public and private schools, and camps. Under the Act, these institutions must, with a few exceptions for religious organizations, make accommodations for a child with diabetes.

Another federal law that relates to children with diabetes is Section 504 of the Rehabilitation Act of 1973. This Act applies to all public, private, and religious schools that receive federal funding. Students with disabilities in addition to diabetes may also be entitled to an Individual Education Plan. These laws also apply to children with type 2 diabetes, although there are many fewer of them, and they tend to be old enough to mostly self-manage their disorder.

The American Diabetes Association makes the following general recommendations for schools:

- Schools should provide trained staff to monitor glucose levels and administer insulin and emergency glucagon injections to counteract hypoglycemia as needed.

- Staff should be trained to recognize the signs of hypoglycemia and hyperglycemia and know how to respond appropriately.

- Trained staff should be available to provide diabetes care during all school-sponsored events, including sports practices, field trips, and overnight trips.

- Schools should allow capable students to self-manage their diabetes. This may mean that the child can carry insulin and a syringe or insulin pen, does not need permission to eat a snack in class, or can leave class to monitor blood glucose or inject insulin.

To facilitate these rights, the ADA strongly recommends that parents provide the school or childcare center with a written Diabetes Medical Management Plan (DMMP) that is created and signed by the child's physician. The DMMP allows the school to legally carry out the orders in the plan, such as giving insulin or treating hypoglycemia. In addition to a DMMP, a written 504 Plan can detail specific actions the school will take to provide support and remove barriers for the diabetic student and ensure appropriate access to the learning environment. For example, a 504 Plan might specify that the child is allowed to eat as needed outside of structured mealtimes; take extra trips to the bathroom; make up instruction missed for medical appointments; and participate in all school-sponsored activities, including sports. Each DMMP and 504 Plan is specific to the individual student and will change as the child's needs change. Sample DMMPs and 504 Plans can be found at https://www.diabetes.org/resources/know-your-rights/safe-at-school-state-laws/written-care-plans.

States also have laws that affect a child with diabetes. At least 34 states and the District of Columbia allow trained teachers, administrators, and coaches to give routine insulin and emergency glucagon injections in accordance with the DMMP and 504 Plan on file for the student. This leaves another 16 states with either incomplete or no laws, while some states have laws that potentially conflict with federal regulations. For example, many schools no longer have a full-time nurse on site, but state law may require that medication be distributed only by a certified health care provider. This can be interpreted to mean that a trained staff member or the student cannot inject insulin at school, a situation that conflicts with the federal requirements to accommodate the child's disability. The ADA provides information on state-specific laws at https://www.diabetes .org/resources/know-your-rights/safe-at-school-state-laws/.

Individual school district policies can also restrict a child with diabetes. Most of these policies concern zero tolerance for possessing medications, weapons, or drugs. Some school districts interpret the possession of a syringe, needle, or insulin pen as a dangerous weapon or as drug paraphernalia. Every year, the Department of Education Office of Civil Rights receives about 45 complaints concerning how school districts fail to follow federal law in accommodating students with diabetes.

A good example of how laws and policies can confound the intention of providing a safe and functional environment for a child with type 1 diabetes was reported in the *Salt Lake Tribune* and the *New York Times* in June 2019. The case involved an eight-year-old boy who needed insulin between four and eight times a day. In kindergarten and first grade, he was given insulin by the school nurse. However, the nurse was not always available when the boy needed the shots, and, on some occasions, he was given the wrong dose of insulin.

The boy's mother, herself a type 1 diabetic, asked if the boy could bring prefilled syringes with the proper dose of insulin, keep them with him at school, and self-administer the insulin as needed. Utah law specifically allows students to carry and self-administer diabetes medication with permission from the child's doctor and a parent.

The problem in this case was that to receive the proper dose for the boy, the standard strength of insulin had to be diluted. His mother, experienced in diluting her own insulin, diluted the insulin and prefilled the syringes at home each day. School district policy, however, allowed medication that was delivered by syringe only if the syringe was prefilled by the manufacturer or a registered pharmacist and labeled by a pharmacist as to its exact content. The school also insisted that the syringes be locked in the administrative office for the safety of other students, despite the fact that school district policy said that "elementary students may carry and self-administer auto injectable epinephrine, insulin, and asthma inhalers during the regular school day" (Tanner 2019), if the proper forms are filed. When the issue concerning prefilled syringes could not be resolved, the family filed a lawsuit to force the school district to comply with what they believe are the disability laws the school is violating. At the time of publication, this lawsuit remained unresolved.

The ADA offers extensive information on the rights of people in the United States with diabetes on their resource page at https://www.diabetes .org/resources. Canadian parents can find information on handling diabetes at school at https://www.diabetesatschool.ca. For U.K. parents, information is at https://www.diabetes.org.uk/guide-to-diabetes/your-child-and-diabetes/schools, and Australian parents can find help at https://www.diabetes australia.com.au/school.

Sports Coaches

Children with diabetes are encouraged to be physically active, because regular exercise increases sensitivity to insulin and appears to improve long-term glucose control as measured by A1c. Many people with type 1 diabetes regularly play sports, swim, run, dance, and participate in other physically demanding activities. Some participate at a professional level. The Americans with Disabilities Act prohibits students with diabetes from being barred from participation in sports at school simply because they have diabetes. It puts the responsibility of having someone available, usually a teacher or coach, who is trained to recognize hypo- and hyperglycemia and respond appropriately.

The situation can be different for sports activities organized by outside groups. In many cases, discrimination laws require a child with diabetes to be included, but the adults organizing outside leagues or clinics tend to be less informed about the disorder. These people may need diabetes education before they feel comfortable taking responsibility for the child and before parents feel safe leaving a diabetic child in their care.

Successfully participating in sports and exercise activities requires that the diabetic match food and insulin to the level and timing of the activity. Extra blood glucose monitoring is needed before and after exercise, as is a heightened awareness of symptoms of hypo- and hyperglycemia. The physician and diabetic management team can help develop a diabetic sports care plan. Guidance from the National Athletic Trainers' Association about what the plan should include can be found at https://type1 .cornerstones4care.com/being-active/growing-up-with-diabetes/playing -competitive-sports.html.

Relatives, Friends, and Babysitters

Most people, especially older people, such as grandparents, have heard of or know someone with type 2 diabetes. These people need to understand that type 1 diabetes is different. Caring for a child with this disorder is more demanding than caring for a person with type 2 diabetes. Not everyone is willing to take on this responsibility, and parents should respect this decision. Those who are willing to become caregivers must understand the child's routine (a written plan is most helpful) and have the skills to monitor blood glucose, give insulin injections if necessary, recognize the signs of hyper- and hypoglycemia, and respond appropriately in an emergency. It usually falls on the parents to do this training, although older children can often manage some self-care.

Diabetes support groups are helpful for finding caregivers who are familiar with type 1 diabetes procedures. These groups can also provide suggestions and support on how to handle questions and problems raised by schools, relatives, friends, and caregivers. A list of support groups by state can be found at https://defeatdiabetes.org/get-healthy/diabetes -support-groups. Diabetes educators can also provide information on local support groups. In addition, information in English and Spanish to help explain and prepare friends, relatives, and others for interacting with a person with type 1 diabetes can be found at https://beyondtype1.org /understanding-type-1-diabetes.

COPING WITH THE WIDER WORLD

The Americans with Disabilities Act requires employers to make reasonable accommodations for people with either type 1 or type 2 diabetes. The Act applies to private employers with 15 or more employees, as well as all state and local government employers. Section 501 of the Rehabilitation Act provides similar protections related to federal employment. Many states have their own laws prohibiting employment discrimination on the basis of disability. These laws limit what an employee must reveal about his or her disability and the health-related questions an employer may ask. Workplace accommodations include adjustments similar to those needed for schoolchildren, such as additional bathroom breaks, time to monitor glucose levels and inject insulin, and adjustments in scheduling. Additional information can be found at https://www.eeoc.gov/laws/types /diabetes.cfm.

Driving, traveling, and developing social and intimate relationships are more complicated for people with type 1 diabetes because the public often lacks awareness of their needs. It can be challenging to educate those in the public unfamiliar with the disorder. Knowing one's rights, along with planning and carrying the proper medical documentation, can smooth the way.

A traveler with diabetes should always carry extra insulin, a glucose monitoring device, injection equipment, glucagon in the event of a hypoglycemic episode, and a backup insulin prescription. Heat above 86°F (30°C), cold below 36°F (2°C), and sunlight cause insulin to break down and become unusable. Insulin must be protected during travel, a power failure, or when a disaster forces hasty evacuation from home.

Airplane travel presents specific difficulties for people with type 1 diabetes. Travelers should request a letter from their doctor explaining their medical need to carry injection devices (sharps), insulin, and juice boxes through security. Insulin pumps and radio-frequency devices used with some glucose monitors can create problems when security personnel are unfamiliar with them. Pumps can safely be worn while passing through metal detection gates, but some manufacturers recommend that people wearing pumps avoid going through body scanners. The pump should never be removed and put through the airport x-ray detector, as this may damage it. Extra time and a pat down are usually required to pass through airport security. A website sponsored by Medtronics at https://www.medtronic diabetes.com/customer-support/traveling-with-an-insulin-pump-or-device gives tips for successfully traveling with diabetes supplies.

Getting a driver's license is a common event that can be complicated by a type 1 diabetes diagnosis. All states have special licensing rules for people with certain medical conditions. Depending on the state, these rules may apply to all people with diabetes or only to those who meet certain conditions, such as using insulin; having a history of hypoglycemic episodes or loss of consciousness; uncorrectable poor vision; or foot damage, such as diabetic neuropathy. In many cases, an additional medical evaluation is necessary to determine if the individual can receive a driver's license. Information on state laws can be found at https://www.diabetes .org/resources/know-your-rights/drivers-licenses-laws. State laws can change, so people should check with their state's licensing agency for the most recent information on medical conditions and driving.

Sex, alcohol, and drugs can play a role in forming social and intimate relationships. Helping friends and potential partners understand the adjustments that must be made can be awkward for all involved. For a person with type 1 diabetes, sex is a physical activity, similar to participation in sports in that it requires adjustments to food and insulin use based on the energy expended. Partners must accept that sex with a type 1 diabetic may not be as spontaneous as with a nondiabetic individual.

Drinking alcohol lowers blood glucose levels and can cause an episode of hypoglycemia. An explanation of the effects of alcohol and ADA guidance on its use can be found in chapter 5, subhead "Alcohol." Hypoglycemia can easily be mistaken for drunkenness in social settings. A person with type 1 diabetes who chooses to drink should inform his or her companions that irrational behavior and slurred speech may indicate a hypoglycemic episode that requires an immediate emergency medical response. Friends should respect diabetic individuals' abstinence or restricted alcohol consumption and never encourage them to have "just one more drink."

Marijuana has been legalized in many states, either for medical or recreational use, but research on how it affects people with type 1 diabetes is scant. As a result, friends may not understand or accept the diabetic individual's choice to abstain from use. One survey discussed in the November 5, 2018 issue of the *Journal of the American Medical Association Internal Medicine* found that individuals who smoked marijuana or consumed marijuana edibles had double the chance of having a life-threatening bout of high blood sugar resulting in diabetic ketoacidosis. Researchers suggested that marijuana use increased appetite. Users consumed more food than normal but, because of the psychoactive effects of marijuana, failed to give themselves the added insulin needed to offset the increased carbohydrates. The study also found that based on A1c readings, regular marijuana users had poorer long-term blood glucose control.

Little research has been done on cannabinoids (CBD). CBD is a marijuana product that is not psychoactive. It has anti-inflammatory properties and is used with varying success to treat pain, seizures, and other health issues. Anyone with type 1 diabetes who wishes to use marijuana or CBD should consult their doctor. The safety picture for using these drugs will likely become clearer as more research is done. The website Beyond Type 1 (https://beyondtype1.org/sex-drugs-diabetes) has guides discussing issues of sex, drugs, and alcohol for people with type 1 diabetes.

EFFECTS OF TYPE 2 DIABETES

Although an increasing number of children and adolescents are now being diagnosed with type 2 diabetes, most people with type 2 are adults capable of treating the disorder without help from others. Management is frequently simplified because they can take oral medication instead of injecting insulin. For those type 2 diabetics who need insulin, concerns about school and workplace discrimination, travel, driving, sex, drugs, and alcohol use are similar to those of people with type 1 individuals, discussed above.

There are fewer studies of how type 2 diabetes affects friends and family than studies of the effects of type 1 diabetes. One study found that people with a type 2 diagnosis, regardless of gender, experience depression after the diagnosis. However, female partners of the diabetic individual also experienced a degree of depression as great or greater than the individual with the diagnosis. Male partners also experience depression, but to a lesser degree than the individual with the diagnosis.

Resistance

Because type 2 diabetes is common, friends and family may fail to recognize that the disorder is serious or that managing it successfully requires lifestyle changes in addition to medication. Family members can help by eating the same healthy diet recommended for the diabetic individual; however, changing adult diets can be difficult, especially with older people who have developed eating patterns over many years. Resentment may develop over dietary changes needed for good glycemic control, especially when one adult in the household wants to continue to buy high-carbohydrate foods that the diabetic should not eat. Type 2 diabetics may hear the same response from family and friends as people trying to lose weight—the "just one treat won't hurt" response.

Unlike type 1 diabetes, which cannot be prevented, type 2 diabetes can often be avoided or moderated through changes in diet and exercise. This is especially true if these changes are made during the prediabetes stage (see chapter 8). Because most people with type 2 diabetes are overweight or obese and few exercise regularly, they are sometimes blamed by family members and acquaintances for having diabetes. Shaming and blaming are not constructive and can increase depression, self-blame, and resistance to compliance. On the other hand, a partner who wants to help by policing everything the diabetic eats is equally unhelpful. Over policing can lead to resentment and bouts of noncompliance.

Blood sugar levels have a strong effect on mood and mood swings. Older individuals with type 2 diabetes tend to be less sensitive to recognizing when their blood sugar is too low or too high. One study found that people with type 2 diabetes had, on average, 19 mild episodes and one serious episode of hypoglycemia each year.

Low blood glucose can cause abrupt mood swings, personality changes, and emotional instability. The individual may become aggressive, angry, or irritable; have bouts of uncontrolled crying; difficulty making decisions; or difficulty concentrating. Conversely, in some people, low blood glucose produces a pleasant feeling of euphoria, almost like being buzzed on alcohol.

High blood glucose can cause nervousness, confusion, and exhaustion. Frequent rapid changes in blood glucose also affect mood. It helps if friends and family are aware that these mood changes may be caused by poor glycemic regulation and can suggest that the diabetic individual check the blood glucose level and take corrective action if necessary.

Diabetes can also place a financial burden on a family. This may cause resentment, especially in high-conflict marriages where partners are critical or hostile to each other or where one partner blames the other for having diabetes. Test strips and other diabetes supplies can be expensive if not covered by insurance (see chapter 5). Resentment can also arise as complications develop, especially sexual complications and those that affect mobility (see chapter 6). Stress arising from conflict with family members often results in poorer glucose control than when partners are knowledgeable and supportive about the disorder.

Some elderly people with type 2 diabetes become forgetful or have dementia and become combative. They are then unable or unwilling to check their blood glucose levels or manage their medication. Others have vision impairments that prevent them from reading their glucose meters, although glucose meters with enlarged numbers and enhanced lighting are available. This puts the burden of medication management on caregivers. Caregivers may cycle through the same emotions as parents of a child with type 1 diabetes, although usually to a less-extreme degree. Patience, a sense of humor, and breaks to prevent diabetes burnout help family members, friends, and caregivers keep resentment and frustration out of their relationships with the diabetic.

8

Prevention

Even though type 1, type 2, and gestational diabetes can produce the same complications, they are very different metabolic disorders. Type 1 and gestational diabetes develop relatively quickly, with few warning signs, and researchers have not found a way of preventing their development. Type 2 comes on gradually. If fasting glucose, oral glucose, and A1c tests are done regularly, the individual has plenty of warning that the disorder is developing and can take steps to prevent or delay its development. Gestational diabetes cannot be prevented, but, as with type 2 diabetes, lifestyle modifications may significantly reduce the risk of it developing or occurring in subsequent pregnancies.

ATTEMPTS TO PREVENT TYPE 1 DIABETES

Type 1 diabetes is an autoimmune disease. The body's immune system, which normally attacks only foreign or sick cells, malfunctions and attacks healthy beta cells in the pancreas. Beta cells are the only source of insulin in the body. Insulin acts as a key that opens a channel into body cells so that they can take in glucose to use as energy. Without insulin, glucose from digested food builds up in the blood. When between 80 and 90 percent of beta cells have been destroyed, the disorder becomes evident. At this point, the individual is likely to develop symptoms of life-threatening DKA (see chapter 5).

Scientists have determined that type 1 diabetes results from a combination of genetic and environmental factors, although they have not pinpointed all the genes or determined which environmental influences trigger the disorder (see chapter 3). However, researchers have devised several clinical trials to test ways of preventing type 1 diabetes, based on what they believe to be the causes. No trials have yet identified a way to prevent the disorder, but they have eliminated some possible triggers and provided clues to others.

Diabetes Prevention Trial—Type 1

The Diabetes Prevention Trial—Type 1 (DPT-1) was a large, multiyear trial begun in 1994. The trial tested whether giving oral or injected insulin to children (median age 10 years) could delay or prevent the development of type 1 diabetes. Participants in the trial all had a close relative with type 1 diabetes. They were given genetic and antibody tests to determine their type 1 diabetes risk. Only those who had a 26–50 percent risk of developing diabetes within five years were included in the trial.

In the oral insulin branch of this trial, participants were randomly assigned to get either a dose of oral insulin or a placebo (inactive substance). Neither the health care professionals administering the trial nor participants knew which group a child was in. Results showed that within a five-year period, both groups developed type 1 diabetes at the same rate. Researchers concluded that it was possible to use genetic and antibody tests to determine a person's five-year risk of developing type 1 diabetes but that giving oral insulin had no effect on the rate of development of the disorder.

In the injection branch of this trial, other participants were randomly assigned to receive either low-dose, long-acting injected insulin twice a day or a placebo. This trial was a complete failure. Sixty percent of children in both the insulin and placebo groups went on to develop type 1 diabetes during the trial period.

Trial to Reduce Diabetes in the Genetically At-Risk

The Trial to Reduce Diabetes in the Genetically At-Risk (TRIGR) looked at the effect of early exposure to cow's milk in infants who were genetically susceptible to type 1 diabetes. The study tested the idea that exposure to the large, complex, foreign proteins in cow's milk early in infancy could trigger the immune system and cause diabetes in susceptible infants. This theory came about through observations that, in the past, type 1 diabetes was not present in Western Samoa or Sardinia, where cow's milk was not used. Yet when cow's milk became available or people from these places moved to areas where cow's milk was used, type 1 diabetes began to show up in children.

Initially, researchers in Canada and Finland fed mice either cow's milk or a formula in which the milk was predigested to make the proteins smaller and undetectable to the immune system. More cow's–milk fed mice developed type 1 diabetes. This supported the idea of a connection between early diet and type 1 diabetes.

The TRIGR study recruited infants in 15 countries who had a close relative with type 1 diabetes and genetic markers that indicated suscepti- bility to the disorder. These infants were breast-fed for four months, and then randomly assigned to be fed for another two months on either a cow's milk formula or a formula in which milk proteins were predigested. They were then followed for a minimum of 10 years to see if there was a difference in the rates at which each group developed diabetes. The study concluded that there was no difference in the development of type 1 dia- betes between the two groups and that avoiding cow's milk would not prevent type 1 diabetes.

European Nicotinamide Diabetes Intervention Trial

Nicotinamide is a form of vitamin B3. It occurs naturally in some foods and is used as a dietary supplement to treat pellagra, a disorder caused by inadequate vitamin B3 that results in skin and mouth inflammation, diar- rhea, and dementia. Nicotinamide is also used to treat acne, and it has been shown to reduce the development of nonmelanoma skin cancers in susceptible individuals. In animal studies, nicotinamide prevented the development of type 1 diabetes. The European Nicotinamide Diabetes Intervention Trial (ENDIT) was designed to test whether nicotinamide could prevent or delay type 1 diabetes in humans.

Individuals from 18 different countries were chosen to participate in this study. They did not have fasting glucose levels that indicated diabetes at the start of the study, but they did have a close relative who had type 1 diabetes. Participants were randomly assigned to receive either nicotin- amide or a placebo for five years. By the end of the study period, 82 people receiving nicotinamide and 77 people receiving the placebo had devel- oped type 1 diabetes. The difference was not statistically significant, and researchers concluded that nicotinamide did not prevent the develop- ment of the disorder.

Diabetes Autoimmune Study in the Young

The Diabetes Autoimmune Study in the Young (DAISY) looked at several different environmental exposures, specifically the time at which solid food was introduced in infant diets, gluten consumption between years one and two, and chronic enterovirus infection. Infants meeting the standard criteria of a close relative with type 1 diabetes and genetic susceptibility participated in this study and were followed to an average age of 13.5 years.

Researchers found that solid food (specifically fruit) introduced before four months or oats and rice introduced after six months appeared to increase the development of diabetes, but these results were not definitive. Breastfeeding concurrent with the introduction of new foods appeared to offer some protection, and nondietary events—specifically, a complicated vaginal delivery—also increased the rate of type 1 diabetes. The rate at which diabetes developed also varied depending on which genetic markers the child had and whether the close relative with the disorder was a mother, father, or sibling.

Overall, the only solid conclusion the researchers could draw was that the safest time to introduce solid food to at-risk infants was between four and five months of age. The DAISY study also looked at gluten consumption throughout the second year of life. Researchers found absolutely no connection between the amount of gluten in the diet during this period and the development of type 1 diabetes.

A different group of researchers in the DAISY study looked at the relationship between enterovirus (stomach virus) infection and type 1 diabetes. In this study, they found no connection between the presence of the virus and diabetes. However, a 2018 review of additional research on a connection between enteroviruses and type 1 diabetes showed strong evidence of a connection and suggested a mechanism by which the virus could trigger, or at least enable, the destruction of beta cells. Currently this avenue of research appears to offer some hope that a type 1 prevention strategy for vulnerable individuals can be developed.

PREVENTION OF TYPE 2 DIABETES

Type 2 diabetes comes with a clear warning flag—a diagnosis of prediabetes. Prediabetes, also called intermediate hyperglycemia, is a condition in which blood glucose levels are higher than normal but are not high enough to meet the diagnosis of diabetes. The American Diabetes Association (ADA) defines prediabetes as a fasting glucose level of 100–125 mg/dl (5.6–7.0 mmol/L), an oral glucose test level of 140–199 mg/dl (7.8–11 mmol/L), and an A1c between 5.7 and 6.4. For many people with prediabetes, type 2 diabetes can be prevented or substantially delayed by lifestyle modifications in diet and exercise and sometimes preventative drug treatment.

Prediabetes—A Call to Action

Eighty-seven million Americans, or about one-quarter of the population, have prediabetes. Half of all people over age 60 are prediabetic. Each year, between 5 and 10 percent of people with prediabetes progress to type 2 diabetes. This results in 70 percent of people with prediabetes eventually developing type 2 diabetes before they die. The first thing a person can do to prevent or delay type 2 diabetes is to have fasting glucose, oral glucose, and A1c tests to determine if they are prediabetic. These are simple blood tests, and yet, 90 percent of people with prediabetes do not know they have the disorder and consequently have no incentive to make the lifestyle modifications that will delay or prevent type 2 diabetes.

The ADA recommends everyone 45 years or older be tested for diabetes. In addition, Asian Americans whose BMI is greater than 23 and anyone else with a BMI greater than 25 and with any additional risk factors should be tested regardless of age. (See chapter 3 for more on risk factors). Some risk factors, such as age, ethnicity, genetic inheritance, and previous gestational diabetes cannot be changed. Risk factors that can be reduced by lifestyle changes include overweight or obesity, smoking, a low level of HDL (good) cholesterol, a high level of triglycerides (fats in the blood), and low physical activity. A brief type 2 diabetes risk test can be found at https://www.diabetes.org/risk-test.

How Type 2 Diabetes Develops

Unlike people with type 1 diabetes, whose ability to make insulin is destroyed, people with type 2 diabetes do make insulin. Yet over time, two things happen. Cells become resistant to insulin, and the amount of insulin beta cells secrete declines.

Insulin secreted into the bloodstream allows cells to absorb glucose. All cells in the body use glucose for energy. Liver, muscle, and fat cells convert and store extra glucose. Over time, a combination of genetic and lifestyle factors can cause body cells to become less sensitive to insulin, a condition known as insulin resistance. The pancreas responds to insulin resistance by making more insulin, but, eventually, beta cells cannot keep up with the demand. They become exhausted, and insulin production decreases. Blood glucose levels rise because cells are no longer able to take in enough glucose to maintain the proper balance in the blood. Initially, this causes few symptoms that the individual would notice. For many people who do not make lifestyle changes, prediabetes develops into type 2 diabetes with all its various complications (see chapter 6).

Prevention through Lifestyle Modification

The lifestyle modifications that can reverse prediabetes, prevent prediabetes from progressing to diabetes, or slow its progression are the same lifestyle modifications recommended for people who already have type 2 diabetes. They are also lifestyle changes recommended by the American Heart Association to help prevent strokes and heart attacks.

The most effective preventative changes that people with prediabetes can make are to increase the amount they exercise and to eat a healthy diet, one that promotes weight loss for those who are overweight. Smokers should quit smoking, and people who drink alcohol should reduce the amount they consume because alcohol damages the liver, and the liver is crucial in storing excess glucose as glycogen.

Exercise increases sensitivity to insulin and improves the ability of muscles to absorb glucose for storage, as well as causing the body to use more glucose for energy. People with prediabetes who have sedentary lifestyles with little physical exertion are encouraged to gradually increase the amount they exercise. Although any amount of exercise is better than none, the minimum amount recommended for Americans ages 18–64 years is 45 minutes five times per week of moderate exercise, such as brisk walking. For Americans over age 65, the minimum is 30 minutes five times per week of moderate exercise, unless restricted by health or mobility. Exercises to increase strength and improve balance are also recommended.

The ADA does not recommend a specific diet. General recommendations are the same as for a heart-healthy diet. To lose weight, individuals must use more calories than they take in. The majority of these calories should come from whole grains, fresh nonstarchy vegetables (carrots instead of corn, for example) and lean meats (e.g., fish, chicken). Consumption of fats should be reduced (e.g., switching from whole milk to 1 percent milk; steaming or baking food instead of frying).

Sugar-heavy foods, such as cakes, pies, sweet rolls, and candy should be eaten only occasionally and in limited amounts. Selecting no-sugar-added processed foods helps eliminate hidden sugar and empty calories. Sugary beverages should be replaced with water, unsweetened tea or coffee, or diet soda. Sugar substitutes generally have no effect on blood glucose but should be used in moderation. Alcohol is high in calories and should be limited. For more diet information, see the dietary guidelines in chapter 5, the Academy of Nutrition and Dietetics website (https://www.eatright.org), or one of the many cookbooks authorized by the ADA or the American Heart Association.

How Well Does Prevention Work?

Multiple studies have found that diet and exercise are effective in reversing prediabetes or preventing its progression to type 2 diabetes. One of the largest, longest, and most intensive study is the Diabetes Prevention Program (DPP) Lifestyle Change study. It began in 1996 at 27 different locations to determine the effectiveness of intensive lifestyle changes, consisting of nutrition education, behavioral self-management strategies, and exercise for preventing type 2 diabetes (group 1). Group 1, called the lifestyle change group, received these services. Group 1 was compared to a group treated with the drug metformin and quarterly education classes (group 2) and a control group that received quarterly education classes and a placebo in place of metformin (group 3). The goal of the program was a 7 percent or greater weight loss, maintenance of that loss, and at least 150 minutes of moderate exercise weekly. The DPP study provided group 1 with lifestyle coaches, intensive counseling and education, group physical activity, and individual strategies for achieving these goals. Forty-five percent of the participants were from minority groups at high risk for developing diabetes.

After three years, participants in the lifestyle-change group (group 1) had lowered their risk of developing type 2 diabetes by 58 percent compared to the control group (group 3). About 5 percent of the lifestyle change group developed diabetes during the three-year period, compared to 11 percent in the control group. Lifestyle change was especially effective in individuals aged 60 and older. This age group reduced their diabetes risk by 71 percent.

The participants in the DPP group taking metformin (group 2) lowered their risk of type 2 diabetes by 31 percent compared to the control group. Metformin was most effective in younger people aged 25–44, women who had previously had gestational diabetes, and people with a BMI of 35 or greater.

After the three-year DPP study, participants were followed for another 15 years. At the 10-year mark, group 1, the lifestyle-change group, continued to have a 34-percent delay in the development of diabetes. Those who did develop diabetes progressed to the disorder four years later than those in the control group 3. Group 2, who continued to take metformin, had an 18-percent delay in the development of diabetes and progressed to the disorder two years later than the control group.

Fifteen years after the active part of the study ended, the lifestyle-change group had a 27 percent delay in the development of diabetes compared to the control group. The metformin group had an 18 percent delay. Overall, 55 percent of the lifestyle-change group and the metformin group had developed diabetes after 15 years, compared to 62 percent of the control group. The National Institute of Diabetes and Digestive and Kidney Diseases, which sponsored the study, concluded that lifestyle changes were both the most health-effective and cost-effective ways to prevent or delay type 2 diabetes.

Other Approaches to Prevention

There is some evidence that intermittent fasting can help prevent prediabetes from progressing or even reverse mild type 2 diabetes. These studies have been small, and it is not clear the degree to which fasting is effective for the general population.

Metformin, a first-line drug used to treat type 2 diabetes (see chapter 5), is sometimes given to prediabetic individuals, especially if they are unable to exercise or have additional health problems. This treatment appears to delay the progression to type 2 diabetes for some people. Several other drugs used to treat type 2 diabetes may also delay its development. However, these drugs often have unacceptable side effects and are less commonly prescribed than metformin. Weight-loss drugs, such as orlistat (Alli, Xenical) may also be prescribed in conjunction with increased exercise and a healthy diet.

Bariatric (weight-loss) surgery (see chapter 5) provides many health benefits to people who are obese and who already have or are at high risk for diabetes and diabetic complications. In some individuals, blood glucose levels return to normal for a significant period after the surgery, and they experience other health benefits, including weight loss and lower blood pressure. For many, however, the decrease in blood glucose is not permanent. A preliminary observational study published in the *Journal of the American Medical Association* in 2019 found that weight-loss surgery in diabetic individuals reduced the risk of serious cardiovascular events and premature death by 50 percent. The surgery is permanent and has some potentially serious complications. People interested in this treatment should thoroughly explore its benefits and risks before undergoing the procedure.

Many studies have looked at the effect of dietary supplements on prevention of type 2 diabetes. In 2019, a review of 83 trials concluded that fish-oil supplements and other omega-3 and omega-6 supplements had no effect on preventing diabetes. As of late 2019, the website https://www .clinicaltrials.gov listed almost 1,000 trials related to supplements for treating prediabetes and preventing type 2 diabetes. To date, there is little reliable information on the use of supplements for diabetes prevention.

Individuals interested in participating in a clinical trial should check the website for trials that are recruiting participants. There is no charge to participate. Participation is free and voluntary. Participants can withdraw from the trial at any time for any reason.

PREVENTION OF GESTATIONAL DIABETES

Gestational diabetes develops in between 2 and 10 percent of pregnant women in the United States. The condition is temporary and resolves after the baby is born, although women who develop gestational diabetes are at higher risk for gestational diabetes during subsequent pregnancies and for the development of type 2 diabetes later in life.

During pregnancy, the placenta makes anti-insulin hormones. This is normal, and, in most cases, the woman compensates by making more insulin. In some women, especially during the late second and third trimesters, anti-insulin hormones overwhelm the amount of insulin the woman can make. When this happens, blood glucose levels rise, and gestational diabetes develops.

The risk of developing gestational diabetes is related to ethnicity, culture, and prepregnancy obesity. The best ways to reduce risk are through diet and exercise, lifestyle modifications that are identical to those used to reduce the risk of type 2 diabetes. Started before pregnancy, these changes appear to have a greater effect in preventing gestational diabetes than the same changes started after pregnancy has been established. One study found that women who had had gestational diabetes could reduce their risk of the disorder occurring during a second pregnancy by 25 percent, but only if lifestyle changes were begun within six months of the first pregnancy and continued until the second pregnancy was complete. Keeping diet and exercise journals has been shown to be more effective than lifestyle-modification education alone.

SERVICE DOGS FOR DIABETICS

In the United States, several organizations such as Dogs for Diabetics, Diabetic Alert Dogs, and 4 Paws for Ability train dogs to detect high and low blood glucose levels and alert their diabetic partners before hypoglycemia or DKA develop. Most people who use diabetic alert dogs have type 1 diabetes, and many of them are children.

Because dogs have a keen sense of smell, they can be trained to recognize chemical changes in the bodies of their diabetic partners that signal either hypoglycemia or hyperglycemia. The dogs are taught to perform a specific behavior when they sense these changes. This behavior alerts the diabetic, who can then take corrective action to prevent hypoglycemia or DKA.

Vision loss is common in people with diabetes, so some service dogs for the blind are cross-trained to act as both guide and diabetes dogs. In the United States, service dogs are permitted to go anywhere the public is allowed, such as schools, restaurants, and on public transportation. Age and other requirements for obtaining a trained diabetes dog vary depending on the program. Costs also vary across different programs.

9

Issues and Controversies

In the United States, issues and controversies surrounding diabetes fall into three categories: political, medical, and legal. Political controversies center on the cost to patients and to society for preventing and treating people with diabetes. Medical controversies involve best practices and the most cost-effective and health-effective ways to manage the disorder. Legal issues are mainly related to the rights of people with diabetes under the Americans with Disabilities Act. They were discussed in chapter 7.

POLITICAL CONTROVERSIES

By 2019, politicians and the public had become increasingly concerned about the rising cost of prescription drugs. Headlines highlighted new immunotherapy drugs that cost hundreds of thousands of dollars to treat a single individual. As eye-catching as these headlines were, the dramatic rise in the cost of insulin affected far more people—people who would die if they could not afford the drug.

The problem of prescription drug costs is primarily a U.S. problem. In countries with single-payer government-managed health care systems, the government directly negotiates drug costs with pharmaceutical companies, and insulin has remained relatively affordable. In the United States, the government's Medicare health plan for people over the age of 65 is the largest payer for insulin. Medicare is, however, barred by law from negotiating drug prices. This condition was written into the original Medicare law as a compromise to get the law passed.

When Insulin Was Not Expensive

The discovery and development of insulin by researchers Frederick Banting and J. R. R. Macleod won them the Nobel Prize in Physiology or Medicine in 1923. Both Banting and Macleod were medical doctors. At the time of their discovery, it was considered unethical for physicians to patent and profit from their medical research. To avoid any conflict of interest, Banting and Macleod assigned the patent for insulin to their coworkers, Charles Best and James Collip, who were not medical doctors. All four researchers agreed to sell the patent for $1 to the University of Toronto where the insulin research had taken place.

The university-owned laboratory soon found that it could not produce enough insulin to keep up with demand, so the patent was licensed to Eli Lilly, a pharmaceutical company in Indianapolis, Indiana. Eli Lilly recognized that access to insulin was the difference between life and death for people with type 1 diabetes and kept the price low and affordable. Even at a low price, the insulin produced large profits. In 1923, the first year that the drug was commercially available, the company sold $1 million worth of insulin—the equivalent of sales of $14.7 million in 2019 dollars. For many years after that, insulin remained financially within reach for most people.

Prices Increase Dramatically

For 50 years, commercial insulin was extracted from pork or beef pancreases. However, in 1983, the FDA licensed the first synthetic human insulin. It was made using recombinant DNA technology (see chapter 2). The research and methods to create synthetic insulin were expensive. The price increased, but the new technology guaranteed a steady supply of insulin because it did not depend on pancreases from slaughtered animals. The laboratory-manufactured human insulin also eliminated the allergic reaction some people experienced with animal insulin. Today, all insulin used in the United States and most other developed countries is produced by recombinant DNA technology.

Between 2002 and 2013, the price of some types of insulin tripled. The cost continued to rise rapidly through 2019, with few signs of slowing. The price increases have caused financial distress for many of the 30 million

Americans who depend on the drug. The uninsured were hardest hit, but even people with insurance felt stressed as co-pays increased. By 2016, the average out-of-pocket costs for a person using insulin, even with health insurance coverage, were $450 per month and were still rising.

Because people with type 1 diabetes make no insulin, they use more of the drug than people with type 2 diabetes, whose bodies usually continue to make some insulin. People with type 1 diabetes generally experience higher-than-average insulin, costs along with the stress of knowing that they can rapidly develop fatal DKA without the drug. As costs rose, many diabetics began skimping on insulin, using smaller doses than they needed for good glucose control or completely skipping doses, thus increasing the chance of serious complications. A small study done at a Yale University diabetes clinic found that one-quarter of their patients were skimping on insulin because of cost.

The Role of Insulin Manufacturers

Three pharmaceutical companies manufacture 90 percent of the world's supply of insulin: Eli Lilly in the United States, Novo Nordisk in Denmark, and Sanofi in France. Because they control most of the supply, these manufacturers are able to influence the price of the drug.

In 2017, a class-action lawsuit filed in Massachusetts claimed that these three manufacturers had colluded among themselves and with pharmacy benefit managers (PBMs) to keep insulin prices artificially high. Since the 2017 suit, other price-gouging lawsuits have been filed, including one by the Minnesota attorney general in 2018. As this book was being written, these cases continued to make their way through the court system.

The big insulin manufacturers seek political influence by spending millions of dollars on lobbyists and by donating to political campaigns. They also make substantial cash donations to nonprofit advocacy organizations, such as the American Diabetes Association (ADA), the Juvenile Diabetes Research Foundation, and the World Diabetes Foundation, a behavior some people consider an unethical attempt to influence research and policy.

The United States uses only 15 percent of the world's insulin but accounts for almost 50 percent of worldwide profits from the drug. In April 2019, Eli Lilly, Novo Nordisk, and Sanofi were required to testify before the United States House of Representatives Energy and Commerce oversight subcommittee to account for their extreme price increases. The only outcome of the hearing was a June 2019 request for more information on pricing.

The Role of Patents

Why is there no generic insulin almost 100 years after the drug was first manufactured? In the United States, since 1995, new drugs are protected by patents for 20 years. However, the basic patent can be extended another five years to make up for the time it takes to get FDA approval to market the drug. Beyond that, there are other relatively simple ways to extend the patent on a drug. Companies can change the way a drug is administered. For example, the same insulin that is given with a syringe gets new patent protection when it is administered by insulin pen.

New patents on old drugs may also be acquired by changing the dosing instructions, making small changes in the drug formula, or even by making changes in the inactive ingredients in the drug. In the case of insulin, small changes to the basic insulin molecule are used to create insulin analogs that alter how fast insulin acts and how long it stays in the body (see chapter 5, Table 5.3 for examples). Each of these insulin analogs creates a new patent.

Since 1980, courts in the United States have also upheld patents on genetically modified organisms, such as the modified bacteria and yeast cells used to produce insulin. Once again, small changes in DNA modifications can be used to acquire a new patent on what is essentially the same drug, because the production process has been slightly changed. All these strategies are legal and are used by drug manufacturers. The result is to prevent or discourage the development of low-cost generic insulin.

The Role of Pharmacy Benefit Managers

Pharmacy benefit managers (PBMs) are companies hired by insurers, corporate employers, health plans, labor unions, and other organizations that offer their members prescription drug benefits. PBMs came into existence around 2002 as a result of changes in Medicare laws. Around the same time, insulin prices started rising.

Physicians associated with PBMs help determine which drugs will be covered by each drug benefit plan. The covered drug list is called the formulary. The drugs included in the formulary vary from insurer to insurer. Listed drugs and patient co-pays change frequently, based on the deals the PBM negotiates.

If a drug is not listed in the formulary, the insurer will not pay for it, and a doctor is unlikely to prescribe it. The threat that a drug may not be listed in the formulary gives PBMs leverage to negotiate discounts off the manufacturer's list price of each drug. PBMs also negotiate rebates from drug companies based on volume sales of specific drugs. Some, none, or all of these discounts may be passed on to the insurer who hired the PBM. The system of discounts and rebates is not transparent to doctors or patients filling prescriptions.

PBMs associate themselves with large networks of retail or mail-order pharmacies, which then become "preferred pharmacies." Preferred pharmacies can fill prescriptions at a lower cost to the patient and with less paperwork than pharmacies not on the preferred list. In exchange for becoming a preferred pharmacy chain, PBMs then charge these pharmacy networks a fee for every prescription that they fill. The fee is based on the list price of the drug, not the actual cost of the drug to the pharmacy, so it is in the financial interest of the PBMs to keep drug list prices high. This arrangement is legal, and it is particularly damaging to people who are uninsured and must pay list price for drugs, such as insulin, that they cannot live without.

In some ways PBMs do help keep some drug costs down. For example, a PBM may require that patients try a lower-cost or generic drug first to see if it is effective before allowing the use of a higher-priced drug to treat the same symptoms. In addition, many specialty or high-price drugs require pre-authorization by a physician who must justify their use. These steps may help hold down the price of some drugs, but overall, since the development of PBMs, patients are paying larger co-pays and have greater out-of-pocket expenses for insulin and many other drugs, even when they have insurance coverage.

Response to Rising Insulin Costs

Insulin manufacturers justify their price increases as necessary to support research and development. In addition, production of insulin is more expensive than manufacturing many other drugs. It involves growing huge amounts of genetically altered bacteria or yeast in climate-controlled fermentation tanks. These cells then secrete insulin into their growth medium, from which it is extracted, purified, and maintained under climate-controlled conditions. However, prices for insulin appear to have risen faster than production costs.

In an effort to offset some of the negative publicity surrounding insulin prices and to discourage government price regulation, Eli Lilly announced in 2019 that it was offering a half-price version of its Humalog insulin. The insulin, identical to Humalog, is called Insulin Lispro and will sell in 2019 for $137.35 per vial. Each vial contains 100 units of insulin. The length of time a vial lasts depends on the individual's daily insulin needs. It will also cap co-pays for insured customers at $95 per month. In response, Novo Nordisk and Sanofi also reduced some prices. Novo Nordisk also announced that beginning in January 2020, it would begin a program to permit diabetics to buy three vials or two packs of insulin pens of certain Novo insulins for a flat cost of $99. This would cover the monthly insulin needs for many diabetics.

Politicians have talked for years about the need to control prescription drug prices but have done little to force change. However, in May 2019, Colorado politicians acted. Starting in January 2020, by law, insured state residents will pay no more than $100 per month in co-pays for insulin, regardless of how much they use. In 2020, Illinois also capped co-pays for its commercially insured residents at $100 for a 30-day supply. At about the same time, the insurer Cigna, which uses Express Scripts as its PBM, announced that it would cap the co-pay of a 30-day supply of insulin at $25, but only if an employer opted into the plan. These are steps in the right direction, but they cover only a small percentage of insulin users and do little for the uninsured.

A Public Relations Controversy

The city of Philadelphia knows that it has a childhood obesity problem. Seventeen percent of its children are overweight, and 22 percent are obese. In 2017, Philadelphia passed a tax of 1.5 cents per ounce on sugar-sweetened and artificially sweetened soft drinks in an effort to reduce childhood obesity. Although the cost of soft drinks rose, obesity rates remained high.

In July 2019, the Philadelphia Health Department followed up with a campaign designed to get parents to stop giving their children sugary snacks. Public service announcements ran on television, online, and on highway billboards that showed a picture of a child eating a doughnut and the words "Today's quick snack could be tomorrow's diabetes."

Parents of children with type 1 diabetes reacted angrily, claiming that the billboards and ads were insensitive and amounted to shaming children whose type 1 diabetes had nothing to do with sugary snacks. The health department responded by adding a sentence to the online and television announcements that read "Prevent T2 Diabetes in Your Kids." The billboards, however, could not be easily altered. This is a local example of how well-meaning attempts to educate about diabetes can cause political controversy and backfire.

MEDICAL CONTROVERSIES

Medical controversies are usually less obvious to patients than political and legal controversies are. They often involve debate about best practices, the prescribing of specific drugs, and concerns about drug interactions. These controversies tend to play out in medical journals and professional association meetings, leaving patients unaware of them.

A1c Regulation

The appropriate target value of A1c in people with type 2 diabetes is one controversy that may directly affect patients. This controversy pits two professional organizations against each other. The American College of Physicians (ACP) released guidance to its members in March 2018 stating that for most people with type 2 diabetes, aggressive medicating to lower A1c values below 7 percent was not in the patient's best interest. (An A1c level of lower than 5.7 percent is considered normal in a nondiabetic person. (See chapter 5 for more details.) The recommendation for an A1c goal of between 7 and 8 percent puts the ACP in direct conflict with the American Diabetes Association (ADA). The ADA has, for many years, recommended that people with type 2 diabetes keep their A1c below 7 percent.

The argument the ACP makes for a higher A1c goal is that it takes about five years for individuals to see health benefits from consistently keeping A1c below 7 percent. Many people with type 2 diabetes are elderly, and the benefits are going to be minimal in their lifetimes. In addition, aggressively medicating with multiple drugs to keep A1c levels below 7 percent increases the chance of experiencing hypoglycemic episodes. The ACP recommends using moderate glucose-lowering drugs along with diet, exercise, and weight management. This approach also treats other health problems that often occur along with diabetes, such as high blood pressure, high cholesterol levels, and obesity. The ACP points out that their approach is a lower-cost option for the patient and reduces the chance of drug interactions and hypoglycemia, which can lead to confusion and falls, especially in older individuals.

The ADA believes that tight glucose control is critical in treating diabetes and its complications. They prioritize glycemic control over treating other conditions that often accompany type 2 diabetes, such as high blood pressure and excessive blood clotting. The ADA believes that tight glucose control and an A1c below 7 percent is almost always in the patient's best interest. They point to several large studies that found the risk of cardiovascular complications and death are reduced at lower A1c levels. These levels, they feel, can and should be achieved through aggressive drug therapy if necessary.

The independence of the ADA's position has been questioned by people who point out that the organization accepts substantial donations from drug companies that make glucose-lowering drugs. This adds a nonmedical element to the debate. In addition, some patients appear to resist the change to a more liberal A1c target, fearing that complications will increase, while others welcome the less stringent targets. It will probably take years and many studies to determine which approach produces the most patient benefits and whether these benefits appear in all type 2 patients or just select subgroups.

10

Current Research and Future Directions

The World Health Organization reported in 2018 that 422 million people worldwide had diabetes. They predicted that soon the disorder would be the seventh-most common cause of death worldwide. These statistics alone provide incentive to prevent, control, or cure diabetes. Despite the fact that, of people with diabetes 95 percent have type 2 diabetes, the most dramatic diabetes research efforts are directed at "solving" type 1, while research on type 2 diabetes often focuses on preventing complications and creating new or improved drugs for glucose control.

TYPE 1 RESEARCH

Research on type 1 diabetes follows several tracks: the creation of an "artificial pancreas"; finding a permanent one-time treatment, often referred to as a "cure" for type 1; and developing ways to delay or prevent onset of the disorder and associated complications. Pharmaceutical companies continue to be interested in developing insulins that act at different speeds and over different periods of time, but this research tends to expand on what is already available rather than offering new approaches to treatment.

The Artificial Pancreas

The artificial or bionic pancreas is not an actual organ but a closed loop, computer-controlled feedback system for automatic insulin administration. Of all the type 1 research currently being undertaken, the artificial pancreas is the closest to becoming approved for everyday use outside of experimental settings.

The goal of the artificial pancreas is to mimic as closely as possible the way a healthy pancreas regulates blood glucose. The system consists of a continuous blood glucose monitor that broadcasts readings to a receiver. The receiver manipulates the information into a useable form and broadcasts it to a smartphone. The smartphone contains an algorithm that calculates the amount of insulin needed to bring glucose levels into the desired range. It then broadcasts the calculation to an insulin pump the individual wears. The pump releases the desired amount of insulin, and the continuous glucose monitor records the change in blood sugar. The process adjusts as necessary every few minutes to keep the individual's blood sugar within the target range. Studies have shown that when a glucagon-like hormone was used in the pump along with insulin, glycemic control substantially improved.

Initially, the artificial pancreas system is given only the individual's weight, but no information about insulin usage, diet, or exercise patterns. Based on the principles of machine learning, the algorithm will then fine-tune or "learn" about the individual's insulin requirements. In hybrid systems, available commercially in 2019, the diabetic individual must program the pump to adjust for meals or changes in activity level. With a fully artificial pancreas, the algorithm makes adjustments to changes in diet and exercise automatically, providing a higher level of freedom for someone with diabetes to eat and exercise without rigorous planning.

As of late 2019, several short-term (several weeks), heavily supervised studies of the artificial pancreas have proved successful. In one study, individuals using the artificial pancreas spent more time in the desired glucose range and had fewer incidents of low blood sugar than when they used a standard insulin pump. The next step is to study long-term use in the real world, without constant physician supervision.

Islet Cell Transplantation

Islet cells are hormone-secreting cells within the pancreas. The two major hormones they secrete are insulin and glucagon (see chapter 1). In type 1 diabetes, healthy insulin-secreting beta cells are destroyed by an out-of-control immune system. Islet cell transplantation is an experimental procedure to replace these destroyed cells.

To perform the transplantation surgery, about four million islet cells are taken from a deceased donor. These cells are then inserted into a vein that goes to the recipient's liver. Over a period of about two weeks, new blood vessels form that connect to established blood vessels in the recipient, and the islet cells begin secreting insulin into the bloodstream. Some researchers are experimenting with enclosing the islet cells in a special coating to protect them from immune system attack. This approach appears promising.

As of late 2019, some islet cell transplantation was in Phase III clinical trials in the United States. Initial results showed that after one year, 90 percent of recipients had A1c values of less than 7 percent, a desirable goal for people with diabetes. About half did not need to take any supplemental insulin. After two years, about 70 percent of people who had undergone transplantation had an A1c level below 7 percent. Forty percent did not need additional insulin. No hypoglycemic events occurred, indicating that the transplanted cells were functioning normally.

Although these results are encouraging, there are some drawbacks. Recipients must take immunosuppressant drugs for as long as the islet cells function in order to prevent their body's immune system from rejecting the foreign cells. This leaves individuals vulnerable to infections. Donor cells are in short supply, and it is not clear how long the donated cells will function. Although not a complete cure, islet cell transplantation has eliminated the need for some insulin injections and improved the quality of life for a significant percentage of recipients with hard-to-control type 1 diabetes. A list of clinical trials currently enrolling patients can be found at https://www.clinicaltrials.gov.

Transforming Cells into Beta Cells

Some very early research has found that, in some cases, an individual's non-beta cells in the pancreas can be converted into beta cells. Researchers in Norway discovered that a small percentage of alpha cells that produce glucagon in the pancreas can be converted into beta cells that produce insulin. The conversion happens through the action of signaling chemicals from surrounding cells. Although only about 2 percent of cells were converted initially, the number can be increased to 5 percent with the application of certain drugs.

In Belgium, researchers are trying to convert a person's liver cells into insulin-producing cells. Cell transformation research is still in a very early stage. However, if the body could make new beta cells, there would be no need to take lifelong immunosuppressant drugs that are required to sustain foreign transplanted islet cells.

Immunotherapy

Type 1 diabetes is an autoimmune disorder, so researchers often look at advances in understanding other autoimmune disorders, such as rheumatoid arthritis, systemic lupus erythematosus, multiple sclerosis, and inflammatory bowel disease, for clues on how to combat type 1 diabetes. One approach that appears to have potential is to block the out-of-control immune system cells that destroy the body's healthy cells.

When a young person is diagnosed with type 1 diabetes, he or she still has as many as 10 percent of functioning beta cells. If the immune system cells that are killing beta cells can be stopped soon after diagnosis, type 1 diabetes may be moderated or perhaps prevented. Interleukin2 (IL-2) is a naturally occurring chemical that helps regulate immune system cells. It is already being used to treat some cancers and has been shown to help moderate other autoimmune disorders, such as systemic lupus erythematosus. IL-2 acts as a signaling molecule to selectively boost the production of certain healthy immune system regulatory cells. The basic idea is to manipulate the immune system so that the "good" immune cells destroy the "rogue" immune cells that damage healthy tissue.

Repurposing an Old Vaccine

Vaccine Bacille Calmette-Guérin, or BCG, was developed in France to treat tuberculosis. It was first used in 1921 and is still used today in countries where tuberculosis is common. In addition to preventing tuberculosis, BCG has other, not easily explainable properties. For example, when injected into the bladder of a person with early stage bladder cancer, the vaccine draws immune system cells to the bladder, where they destroy cancer cells.

BCG appears to boost the production of a signaling molecule called tumor necrosis factor (TNF). In people with autoimmune diseases, TNF can destroy the rogue immune system cells that attack healthy body tissue, such as islet cells. Researchers believe that BCG somehow helps reset the immune system back to normal and, thus, controls autoimmune disease. The vaccine has been used experimentally to treat people with multiple sclerosis, another autoimmune disease, with promising results.

In experimental results shared at the American Diabetes Association (ADA) scientific conference in 2018, researchers reported that they had injected an experimental group of people who had been diagnosed with type 1 diabetes for a minimum of two years (many had been diabetic for more than a decade) with BCG twice, four weeks apart. The average A1c at the beginning of the study was 7.36 percent (less than 7.0 is generally the goal for diabetics). Although no reduction in A1c was observed during the first three years after BCG injection, the average A1c fell to 6.1 after five years and was 6.6 at eight years. Controlling A1c is considered necessary to prevent diabetic complications. The importance of these results is that two doses of vaccine worked in people who had long-standing diabetes and continued to work over a long period.

TYPE 2 RESEARCH

Research on type 2 diabetes centers on developing a better understanding of who is at risk of developing the disorder and experimenting with the most effective prevention and education messages to help people prevent type 2 diabetes and its complications. To date, psychology and public health researchers have found it difficult to craft a message that will make people change their diets and exercise habits. Pharmaceutical companies continue to search for profits by developing more effective drugs that allow better glucose control with fewer side effects and heavily advertising these drugs. Other areas of research are very new. Many are intriguing but have not yet reached the human-testing stage.

Restoring Beta Cell Function

Unlike people with type 1 diabetes, people with type 2 diabetes still have beta cells. Although the beta cells have not been killed, their insulin output has diminished to the point where it no longer maintains glucose control. A Swedish research team believes that these poorly producing beta cells can be restored by blocking a protein called VDAC1 that is found in beta cells. When this protein accumulates, it affects cellular metabolism. If a substance that blocks the formation of this protein is given to people with prediabetes or early type 2 diabetes, the researchers believe that beta cells will continue to function, and diabetes may be prevented. Successful animal studies have been conducted, but, as of 2019, no human studies had been undertaken.

Modifying the Microbiome

The microbiome is all the bacteria and viruses that live on and within us. In recent years, researchers have found that the microbiome of the gut plays a significant role in health. Abnormal microbiomes have been linked to inflammatory bowel disease, multiple sclerosis, and cancer. An individual's microbiome is affected by diet, age, exercise patterns, and location. People with type 2 diabetes have been found to have a less diverse microbiome than healthy people. This opens up the possibility that balancing the microbiome may help prevent diabetes.

As of 2019, one company in France has transplanted fecal matter containing the biome of a healthy gut into obese diabetics. This procedure produced a short-term improvement in insulin resistance. Because diabetics have a less diverse biome than nondiabetics, another company is focusing on therapies that increase the diversity of the gut biome. This area of research is quite new and complex, but it could hold clues as to why some people develop type 2 diabetes, while others do not, and it suggests novel ways to prevent or treat the disorder.

New Drugs and New Delivery Systems

Since 2010, at least 40 new drugs to treat diabetes have been approved by the Food and Drug Administration. One can hardly turn on the television without seeing advertisements for these drugs (see chapter 5). Some drugs target beta cells to stimulate them to produce more insulin. Others target muscle, fat, and liver cells that take up excess glucose. By 2025, the market for diabetes treatments is expected to exceed $95 billion (€86 bn), so pharmaceutical companies continue to work toward new drugs that provide better blood glucose control with fewer side effects. At least one drug under development will treat high blood pressure along with diabetes, since the two conditions are often found together.

A growing number of people with type 2 diabetes need to take supplemental insulin by injection to prevent hyperglycemia. An oral pill would be preferable to injection and would likely improve compliance. In 2017, Novo Nordisk abandoned the development of a long-acting oral insulin pill, even though it was as effective as the long-acting injectable insulin glargine. However, in 2018, another company began a small clinical trial in New York of an oral insulin tablet that was enclosed in a protective coating to prevent it from being destroyed by acid in the stomach.

Finally, in 2019, a group of researchers at the Massachusetts Institute of Technology and Novo Nordisk developed an oral device containing insulin. The tiny device was constructed so that it always positioned itself in a specific alignment against the stomach wall and remained there, even if the stomach moved and contracted. Once in position, a microneedle made of freeze-dried insulin is injected into the stomach wall. From there, the insulin is absorbed into the bloodstream. As of 2019, this device had been used successfully in animals but had not been tested in humans.

Better Glucose Monitoring

Finger sticks to measure blood glucose are a significant annoyance, and many people with type 2 diabetes are tempted to skip them. Research is underway to find easy, noninvasive ways to get accurate blood glucose readings. It is believed that such methods will encourage people to check their glucose levels more frequently and encourage medication compliance.

A device that uses electromagnetic waves to measure glucose is already available in Europe, and devices that measure glucose using laser light or radio waves are also under development. Readings are then sent to a receiver or smartphone, where they are available to the individual and can be uploaded to a computer or to the cloud.

Patches and implantable devices for measuring glucose are currently available, but there is a move toward making these devices smaller, less costly, and longer lasting. For example, a Dutch company is working on a tiny glucose-measuring device that would be implanted under the eyelid. Not all these devices will make it to market. Google's glucose-measuring contact lens, for example, went nowhere. But the goal of all these devices is to make measuring and controlling blood glucose simpler and more convenient. The hoped-for result is better medication compliance and a reduction in the complications of diabetes.

Case Illustrations

EMMA COPES WITH A MISUNDERSTANDING

Emma developed type 1 diabetes when she was five years old. When she was 15, her family moved, and she enrolled in a new high school. Just as they had done at her old school, Emma's parents met with school officials and discussed her medical needs and her rights under the Americans with Disabilities Act. They came to an agreement with the school about specific actions the school would take related to Emma's health and education. These actions were recorded in a Section 504 Plan, as authorized under the Rehabilitation Act of 1973. In addition, the parents provided the school with a physician-approved Diabetes Medical Management Plan. It provided additional medical and contact information and allowed the school to legally give Emma insulin or treat her for hypoglycemia.

State law and school district policy allowed Emma to carry an insulin pen at school and to inject herself, something she had been doing for several years. Accommodations agreed to in the 504 Plan included allowing Emma to leave class to check her blood glucose level or inject herself with insulin, to eat at nonstandard times to prevent hypoglycemia, and to take water and bathroom breaks as needed. Because Emma was experienced in managing her diabetes and did not want to call attention to herself in her new school, she rarely used the 504 provisions.

One day, however, during a geometry test, Emma started sweating even though the room was cool. She felt shaky. Her head ached. She recognized that these were signs that her blood sugar was too low. She needed to eat something containing sugar immediately.

Not wanting to disturb the other test takers, Emma quietly left the classroom. She went as planned to the school office, since the school did not have a full-time nurse. There she was given a private place to check her blood glucose level, which was too low. To correct this, she ate several glucose tablets that she kept with her for emergencies. When she felt better, she checked her glucose level. It was within the normal range, so she returned to class.

The period was almost over, and Emma was only able to complete two geometry problems. She handed in what she had done and hurried off to her next class, without explaining to the teacher why she had left class. The next day, her test was returned with a failing grade. After school that day, she went to see the teacher.

"I have diabetes," Emma explained. "I left class because I started to feel shaky and needed to check my blood sugar level."

"You mean you can just get up and walk out of class any time you want?" the teacher asked. "That doesn't sound right to me. It seems like any time you have a test you don't want to take, you can simply leave and claim you did not feel well. Why couldn't you wait until class was over?"

"I've learned to recognize when I'm hypoglycemic. If I don't get some sugar in me right away, I get disoriented. Once, I had seizure and passed out."

"My aunt has diabetes, and she never has to drop everything and eat," the teacher said. "I think you're taking advantage of your condition."

Emma sighed. She often had to deal with people who did not realize that type 1 and type 2 diabetes were different disorders or who did not realize how quickly serious complications could develop for people with type 1 diabetes.

When the teacher refused to allow her to take a make-up test, Emma went to the assistant principal and explained her situation. The assistant principal called a meeting between Emma, the teacher, and Emma's mother. He explained to the teacher that Emma had a legitimate disability that gave her certain rights, one of which was to leave class when she felt her health was endangered. The teacher did not like being corrected. She insisted that Emma was wrong to simply leave class without an explanation, but she grudgingly said she would let Emma take a make-up test. The principal agreed that Emma should have spoken to the teacher before leaving. He instructed Emma that in the future, she should tell her teachers about her condition before leaving class. Emma was not happy with this requirement. She did not want her classmates to know she had diabetes or to be singled out as different.

Analysis

Emma was correct that hypoglycemia is a serious condition that needs immediate attention. Her parents had filed all the correct paperwork and made an effort to educate school officials about Emma's condition. She had the right and the school administration's permission under her 504 Plan to leave class to check her blood glucose level and to take steps to correct it or seek medical help.

Where the school failed was in not informing teachers of Emma's situation. This could have simply been an oversight or an attempt to protect Emma's privacy, as certain laws prevent the sharing of medical information. The absence of a school nurse complicated the question of who should be told about Emma's diabetes.

Emma did not help her situation by leaving class without explaining why, especially when taking a test. Like many teenagers with type 1 diabetes, Emma did not want to call attention to her disorder for fear that other students would either avoid her or pity her. In her old school, which she had attended since kindergarten, her friends had grown up accepting that she had special health needs. Afraid of the judgment of students in her new school, Emma tried to hide her disorder to seem as much like her nondiabetic peers as possible. This contributed to the teacher's failure to understand why Emma had left class, but it did not excuse the teacher's refusal to let Emma take a make-up test once she had explained her condition.

ROGER LOSES HIS FOOT

Roger had been physically active and in good shape for most of his life. For years, he worked in construction but was forced to quit when a rotator cuff injury caused weakness and pain in his right shoulder. For the next five years, Roger worked as a security guard at a factory. He spent much of his time sitting in a guard booth at the main gate, checking people and vehicles in an out.

Even though Roger now spent hours sitting instead of doing physically demanding work, he continued to eat the way he had when he was a construction worker. He enjoyed large meals that were heavy on meat, potatoes, or pasta, and he never missed dessert. Every day at lunch, he drank a soda with his sandwiches, and on most evenings, he had a couple of beers and snacked on chips in front of the television. Not surprisingly, he gained weight, and by the time he was 62 and went for a physical, he weighed 48 pounds more than when he had when he worked construction.

As part of his physical, Roger had a fasting blood glucose test. It showed a reading of 118 mg/dl. Other blood work showed that he had high cholesterol and high triglycerides.

"You have prediabetes," the doctor said.

"What does that mean?" Roger asked.

"It means that there is a good chance you will develop diabetes."

"How good a chance?" Roger asked. "What are the odds?"

"That depends on you. If you get more exercise, eat a healthy diet, and lose some weight, you can significantly reduce your diabetes risk."

"Okay. Okay," Roger said.

He took the information on diabetes that the doctor gave him. At home, Roger tossed it in the trash and soon forgot about what the doctor had said. He continued to drink soda and beer, snack on chips and cookies, and gain weight. He occasionally felt guilty and promised himself that he would start exercising and eating better, but he never did. He was embarrassed that he hadn't lost weight, so he avoided annual physicals.

Over the next few years, Roger often felt tired and had to get up several times each night to urinate. His feet often felt cold and numb. He thought these annoyances were part of normal aging.

One day when Roger put on his socks, he noticed a blister on the ball of his foot. It didn't hurt much, so he ignored it. A few weeks later, the blister had become an open sore. The sore was not particularly painful, but after about six weeks, it was still there. Roger decided this was not normal and made an appointment to see a podiatrist.

The podiatrist told Roger that he had a diabetic foot ulcer. He referred Roger to a diabetes specialist and a vascular surgeon to evaluate the blood flow in Roger's legs. This seemed to Roger like a lot of fuss over something that did not bother him all that much. He put off making the appointments, but the wound still did not heal.

When Roger eventually saw the specialists, he was shocked to learn that the tissue in his foot was dying because of lack of blood flow, a condition called gangrene. Because of this, the gangrenous tissue would have to be surgically removed, and Roger would need vascular surgery to try to improve blood flow to the foot to stop more tissue from dying. Roger finally realized the seriousness of his diabetes and of his foot wound.

The gangrenous tissue was removed, but vascular surgery was unsuccessful in restoring adequate blood flow to prevent more tissue death. The only way to stop gangrene from spreading was to amputate the foot. The amputation was successful, but Roger lost the ability to walk and now uses a wheelchair.

Analysis

Type 2 diabetes, although extremely common, can cause serious complications. When Roger was diagnosed as prediabetic, the doctor explained how he could reduce his risk of developing type 2 diabetes. Roger ignored the advice and did not change his eating and exercise habits. Since he had no symptoms of illness when he was diagnosed with prediabetes, the possibility of developing diabetes seemed minor and far off—something he could deal with in the future.

Type 2 diabetes develops slowly. Fatigue; excessive thirst and increased urination; blurry vision; and cold, numb, or tingling feet or hands are all symptoms of the disorder, but they are often explained away as just part of aging. Roger ignored these symptoms, and because he avoided going to the doctor, he became one of the 8.1 million Americans whose diabetes remained undiagnosed and untreated.

Diabetic ulcers like the one Roger experienced on his foot often are not painful because years of uncontrolled high blood glucose have damaged nerves in the feet, a condition called diabetic neuropathy. These wounds do not heal because high blood glucose also damages the blood vessels in the feet and legs. As a result, the foot ulcer did not receive enough oxygen and nutrients to heal.

People with diabetes need to inspect their feet regularly and see a health care professional as soon as they notice any damage. Had Roger realized he had diabetes, he might have sought care for his foot wound early, and then steps could have been taken to save his foot. These include daily care of the wound, special footwear, hyperbaric oxygen treatment, and surgery to reduce pressure on the wound. The likelihood of Roger losing his foot would have been significantly reduced if he had taken his diagnosis of prediabetes seriously and made lifestyle changes, learned the symptoms of type 2 diabetes, and seen a doctor when he developed a wound that would not heal on its own.

MARIA ROSA DEVELOPS GESTATIONAL DIABETES

Maria Rosa, a 28-year-old Latina, was excited to be pregnant with her first child. Although she was moderately overweight at 170 pounds (77 kg), with a BMI of 27.4 when she became pregnant, her pregnancy progressed normally until the 24th week, when she was given a routine fasting glucose test for gestational diabetes. The test came back with a glucose reading of 130 mg/dl (7.2 mm/L), and a repeat test was slightly higher.

"This test shows that you have gestational diabetes," the doctor told Maria Rosa.

"Diabetes? But I feel fine," Maria Rosa said. "Why would I get diabetes now?"

"This type of diabetes is related to your pregnancy. Soon after the baby is born, it should go away."

The doctor then explained that during pregnancy, it is normal for the placenta to produce hormones that make the cells in the body more resistant to insulin. "Your body is not making enough insulin to overcome these pregnancy hormones, so too little glucose is entering cells," he told Maria Rosa. "When this happens, the amount of glucose in the blood increases, and this can be damaging. The test you had tells us that the level of glucose in the blood is too high."

The doctor sent Maria Rosa home with a diet and exercise plan as the first step in trying to lower her blood glucose. "But," she told Maria Rosa, "when you come in for your retest next week, if your glucose is not back to normal, we will need to start you on insulin."

Maria Rosa followed the diet and exercise program, but the following week, her glucose level was still too high, so the doctor started her on insulin and showed her how to check her blood glucose level at home. Maria Rosa was stunned that she would have to inject herself twice a day. She had imagined that the doctor might prescribe pills, but taking shots made her gestational diabetes seem much more serious. She worried that the baby might have a birth defect because of her diabetes. The doctor assured her that gestational diabetes did not increase the risk of birth defects or miscarriage.

Maria Rosa learned to inject herself with insulin, and faithfully checked and recorded her blood glucose level several times each day. She made an effort to eat well and to increase her activity level. At one appointment, her blood pressure was elevated. The doctor was concerned, but the increase was temporary and never rose into the danger zone.

Maria Rosa kept all her medical appointments. She wanted a healthy baby. As her due date approached, the doctor determined that she was going to have a very large baby. This is common in women with gestational diabetes.

"It looks like your baby is going to weigh around 10.5 pounds (4.5 kg)," the doctor said. "It would be best of we deliver your baby by a scheduled cesarean section. Babies this large can be damaged when they are forced through the birth canal, and the mother's tissues can be torn. It is better to schedule a cesarean than to have an emergency one if you have an unsuccessful labor."

Maria Rosa had a baby girl by cesarean section. As soon as the baby was born, she was whisked away to the neonatal intensive care unit (NICU) because she was experiencing seizures caused by hypoglycemia. In the NICU, she was treated with intravenous glucose, and, in a few days, she was healthy and ready to go home. At discharge, Maria Rosa was told there was a high probability that she would have gestational diabetes with future pregnancies and that she had an increased risk of developing type 2 diabetes in the future. She was also reminded to return in two to three months for another fasting glucose test to make sure her gestational diabetes was gone.

Analysis

Gestational diabetes occurs in about 10–15 percent of pregnancies, although it is not evenly distributed across ethnic groups. Latina, Native American, and African American women have much higher rates of gestational diabetes than Caucasian women. Maria Rosa had several risk factors for the disorder. She was a Latina. She was over the age of 25. She was overweight when she became pregnant and experienced rapid weight gain during pregnancy.

When given a fasting glucose test, Maria Rosa's blood glucose was above 126 mg/dl (7.0 mm/L). Any reading higher than this is a diagnosis of diabetes. In Maria Rosa's case, the diabetes was directly related to her pregnancy. Her blood glucose level should decrease to normal levels by about six weeks after the baby's birth. However, having had gestational diabetes, she is at higher risk for developing type 2 diabetes and should have a fasting glucose test every one to three years to make sure that type 2 diabetes has not developed. Later in life, Maria Rosa's daughter may also have an increased risk of developing type 2 diabetes or gestational diabetes.

The baby was taken to the NICU because she was experiencing hypoglycemia. This occurs in up to one-third of babies born to mothers with gestational diabetes. It happens because the baby's pancreas begins making insulin in the womb to cope with the high level of glucose in the mother's blood. When the baby is born and is no longer exposed to the mother's blood, his or her glucose levels drop rapidly, but, for a brief time, the baby's pancreas continues to make insulin. During this period of excess insulin production, hypoglycemic can occur.

Hypoglycemia in newborns can be very serious and can cause seizures, coma, and even death. Promptly treating the baby with intravenous glucose prevents these complications. In a few days, the baby's pancreas will adjust its insulin production, and the baby will be healthy.

SHANTAL TAKES PREVENTATIVE ACTION

Shantal is a 33-year-old African American woman. She is seriously overweight, with a BMI of 29.5, but is otherwise in good health. As an administrative assistant, she spends much of her day sitting at a desk. Her only regular exercise is a short walk to the bus stop each morning. Shantal loves to bake and often brings treats she's made to the office. On many weekends, she cooks for her extended family when they get together to play cards and watch sports.

Shantal went to the doctor for her annual physical. Because she had some risk factors for type 2 diabetes—African American ethnicity, a BMI greater than 25, and an inactive lifestyle—the doctor ordered a fasting blood glucose test. The result indicated that Shantal had prediabetes. Her blood glucose was higher than normal, but not high enough to diagnose diabetes.

"You are quite young to have prediabetes," the doctor said. "Most people who develop prediabetes at your age progress to type 2 diabetes."

Shantal told the doctor that diabetes ran in her family. Her sister had gestational diabetes with both her pregnancies. At least two of her cousins took medicine for diabetes. Her Uncle Charles, who was only 59, had had diabetes for years but had never taken his condition seriously. He skipped doctor appointments, refused to check his blood glucose, and rarely took the medicine the doctor prescribed. Now he had kidney disease and was on the waiting list for a kidney transplant. While he waited, his wife had to take him for dialysis three times a week. The aunt had quit her job in order to care for Charles, and Shantal knew she was stressed by the loss of income and fearful that Charles would die before a suitable kidney could be located.

"I feel like this is a curse on my family, and there is nothing I can do," Shantal said.

"That's not true. It is not inevitable that you will develop diabetes," the doctor said. "If you are willing to change your diet and get more exercise, you may be able to reverse the prediabetes. Even if you can't, those changes will likely delay the development of full-blown type 2."

The doctor gave Shantal some written information and encouraged her to attend a diabetes education class that the hospital offered at night. She also advised her to make an appointment with a diabetes nutritionist or a diabetes educator, reminding her that their services were covered by her health insurance.

It took Shantal a few weeks to come to grips with the idea that she was going to have to make changes in her life if she wanted to avoid the fate of her cousins and uncle. Eventually, she went to the evening class and learned how healthy eating and exercise could reduce her blood glucose level. She even made an appointment with the nutritionist.

"It's great that you like to cook," the nutritionist said, handing Shantal a collection of healthy recipes. "So many people I see live on fast food. When they do cook, they prepare highly processed foods, but since you're an experienced cook, you won't have any trouble preparing healthy meals."

That made Shantal feel a bit better about herself. Healthy meals were something she knew she could do, but she wasn't happy about needing to get more exercise. At the diabetes class, the instructor encouraged people to join a gym to get regular exercise. Shantal knew there was no way she was going to work out in a gym. She was self-conscious about her weight and could not face the idea of exercising in public.

"Walk," the diabetes instructor said when some had asked about alternatives to a gym. "Walk briskly at least 30 minutes per day." Shantal figured she wouldn't mind walking more. She bought a pair of comfortable walking shoes and started passing by the nearest bus stop and walking to the next one on the line each day. At first, she resented the time this took, but eventually she came to appreciate that the walk was more than exercise. It gave her a chance to de-stress from work each day, and she felt more relaxed when she got home.

It has been three years since Shantal started her diet and exercise program. Several months passed before she saw consistent results, but, today, her blood glucose level hovers at the high end of normal. She still cooks for her family when they get together, but now she serves more vegetables and fewer fried foods, and she has lost 14 pounds without conscious dieting.

Analysis

Shantal was fortunate that her prediabetes was diagnosed so early. Many people have prediabetes or type 2 diabetes and do not know it because symptoms come on gradually and are often attributed to other causes. In addition, she was motivated to change her habits because she had seen in her own family how damaging type 2 diabetes could be.

Although it did take her a while to accept that she had to change, once Shantal got used to the idea, she got information and professional help from a diabetes educator and nutritionist. From them, she learned that diet alone probably would not reduce her blood glucose. She also needed to exercise because exercise would make muscles use more glucose and make cells less resistant to insulin. Once insulin resistance was reduced, more glucose could enter cells instead of staying in the blood.

A big reason Shantal was successful in sticking with her diet and exercise program was because she found ways to work her new habits into activities she enjoyed. She still loved cooking, but she no longer made as many cookies and pies and concentrated instead on finding tasty ways to cook vegetables and lean meats.

Like many overweight people, Shantal was uncomfortable with the idea of exercising at a gym, where other people would notice her. Instead, she found a way to add regular walking to her routine. Her blood glucose might have decreased faster and she may have lost more weight by going to the gym, but, more importantly, she found a successful program she could incorporate into her life and stick with for years.

JACKSON'S WIFE RESENTS HIS DIABETES

Jackson is 74 years old. He was diagnosed with type 2 diabetes 16 years ago. When he was diagnosed, his wife, Charlotte, resented that she needed to change the way she cooked. Many of the foods she made regularly were not good for Jackson, but she resisted experimenting with new, healthier dishes. She often made foods that she liked but were poor choices for Jackson and insisted that a small helping would not hurt him. Jackson found it hard to stay on a healthy diet, especially since Charlotte still brought home cookies and ice cream from the store that tempted him. Consequently, Jackson's blood glucose was often too high. Within several years, he progressed to needing insulin injections. He had difficulty managing his insulin dosage and sometimes had scary hypoglycemic episodes.

For a few years after his diagnosis, Jackson's vision did not change noticeably, but, gradually, his sight deteriorated. When he went to the ophthalmologist, he learned that he had severe nonproliferative retinopathy and that it was likely to progress until he became blind. At this news, he became depressed and, for several months, made little effort to exercise or control his diet.

Eventually Jackson did lose his sight. This made him heavily dependent on his wife. He became seriously depressed, and she became short-tempered and frustrated because his blindness put all the responsibility for his care, the house, shopping, and driving on her just as she was growing older and having some health problems of her own. The situation in their house was tense and unhappy.

The ophthalmologist recommended that Jackson enroll in an orientation and mobility program offered by the local hospital. This helped build his confidence and made him better able to care for himself. Through the orientation and mobility program, Jackson learned that he could apply for a "seeing eye," or guide dog. He applied to several organizations that train dogs for the blind. During the application and interview process, he discovered that some guide dogs were cross-trained as diabetic alert dogs. These dogs learn to recognize a scent that a person with low blood sugar gives off, and then execute a specific behavior, or alert, to warn the person that he or she is close to having a hypoglycemic episode.

Jackson was accepted into a program that cross-trained dogs. It took him several months of daily training to learn to trust that the dog would keep him safe, but once the pair bonded, Jackson and the dog could walk and travel on public transportation independently. This took some of the pressure off Charlotte and helped restore some of Jackson's social life.

Even though his mobility had improved, Jackson continued to have problems with hypoglycemic episodes; however, with a cross-trained diabetic alert dog, he avoided any serious episodes. As Jackson and the dog bonded, his depression lifted, and the atmosphere at home became less tense. With the easing of tensions, Jackson became more conscientious about following his diet, exercise, and medication program, and his glycemic control improved.

Analysis

Diabetes is a disorder that affects not just the diabetic but friends and family as well. Some family members resent the changes they must make to accommodate the diabetic. Jackson's wife had cooked the same way for many years. Learning a new way of thinking about food and nutrition took her out of her comfort zone, and she resented this. It is not uncommon for family members to interfere with the diabetic's need to develop new eating habits.

Diabetes distress, a collection of negative emotions that include depression, anxiety, stress, frustration, and anger, is common in people diagnosed with diabetes. In addition to health worries, diabetes treatment can be a financial burden and can change the balance of responsibilities in a household. Rapid mood swings are common in people, like Jackson, who have difficulty controlling their blood glucose levels, which can add to household stress. Studies show that spouses often experience the same negative emotions as the person with diabetes. It is not surprising that tensions arose between Jackson and Charlotte.

Once Jackson could no longer see well enough to draw up the correct dose of insulin into a syringe, Charlotte had to take on this job, along with all the other responsibilities that went with caring for someone who was newly blind. Over time, she likely experienced periods of resentment and caregiver burnout, while Jackson may have felt guilty about the effect his diabetic complications had on Charlotte.

The orientation and mobility program Jackson attended helped improve both his life skills and his feeling of having some control over his disability. Getting a guide dog gave him even more control. As he came to trust the dog, his ability to go places on his own increased. This took some of the burden off Charlotte. It also gave him the opportunity to socialize without her assistance. The fact that the dog could alert Jackson to an impending bout of hypoglycemia made him more aware of the need take responsibility for controlling his blood sugar. Slowly, the tension between Jackson and Charlotte eased, as they adjusted to the changes in their life.

Glossary

Agonist
A drug that acts on cells to cause a specific action to occur.

Alpha cell
A type of cell in the pancreatic islets that releases the hormone glucagon when blood glucose levels fall below the normal level. This stimulates the liver to break down stored glycogen into glucose and release it into the bloodstream.

Amylin
A hormone secreted by beta cells in addition to insulin. It slows the production of glucagon and also slows stomach emptying to help prevent glucose spiking after meals.

Antagonist
A drug that acts on cells to block a specific action or reduce its effect.

Antibody
A protein molecule produced in response to a specific antigen in order to destroy the cell carrying the antigen.

Antigen
A nonself molecule that stimulates an immune system response that results in the production of antibodies.

A1c Test
A simple blood test that measures the percentage of hemoglobin to which glucose is attached in red blood cells. The A1c reading is an average over about a three-month period and does not reflect day-to-day glucose readings. The higher the concentration of glucose over time, the higher the A1c. This test is sometimes called a hemoglobin A1c (HbA1c) test.

Arteriosclerosis
The thickening and hardening of the walls of arteries that results in a loss of elasticity.

Atherosclerosis
The narrowing of arteries that results from buildup of waxy plaque on the interior artery walls. This often follows the development of arteriosclerosis.

Autoimmune Disorder
A disorder that occurs when the immune system malfunctions and attacks healthy body cells. Examples include type 1 diabetes, multiple sclerosis, and rheumatoid arthritis.

Basal Dose
The dose of insulin needed to keep glucose levels in the desired range between meals.

Beta Cell
The major type of cell found in pancreatic islets. Beta cells secrete insulin into the bloodstream. Insulin allows glucose to be used in the body. If beta cells are damaged or destroyed and not enough insulin is produced, a person develops diabetes. Beta cells also secrete the hormone amylin but in much smaller quantities than insulin.

Body Mass Index (BMI)
A weight-to height ratio used to define conditions of being underweight (below 18.5), normal weight (18.5–24.9), overweight (25.0—29.9), or obese (30.0 or greater). Overweight or obese BMIs are a reason to have blood glucose levels tested.

Bolus Dose
A dose of medicine given at a single time. In diabetes, it refers to the amount of insulin given before meals to cover the amount of carbohydrates in the food that will be eaten.

Cirrhosis
An irreversible liver disease characterized by loss of liver cells and scarring.

Clinical Trial
A research study using humans in which volunteers are assigned to various groups to test the safety and effectiveness of a new drug or treatment before it is licensed for public use.

Diabetic Ketoacidosis (DKA)
A condition that arises when inadequate insulin prevents glucose from entering cells so that blood glucose levels are high. Fat broken down to use as alternative energy creates molecules called ketones, which cause the blood to become acidic. The condition can be fatal.

Electrolytes
Salts and minerals that ionize in body fluids. Electrolytes control the fluid balance of the body and are important in muscle contraction, energy generation, and almost all major biochemical reactions.

Fasting Blood Glucose Test
A simple blood test performed after fasting for eight hours that measures the amount of glucose in the blood. The result can determine if a person has diabetes.

Gangrene
Tissue death due to lack of blood circulation or infection. If not controlled, gangrene can spread through the body and cause death. It is the leading cause of limb amputation in diabetics.

Glucagon
A hormone secreted by alpha cells in the pancreas that signals the liver to break down glycogen into glucose and release it into the bloodstream when blood glucose levels are too low.

Glucose Spiking
A sharp rise in blood sugar after eating.

Glycogen
A stored form of glucose made by linking several glucose molecules together.

Glycosuria
Sugar in the urine; a symptom of untreated diabetes.

Hemoglobin
The molecule in red blood cells that carries oxygen to all parts of the body. Glucose attaches to some hemoglobin molecules in red blood cells. Measuring the amount of hemoglobin attached to glucose with an A1c test gives information about average glucose levels over about three months. The three-month limit occurs because that is the life span of individual red blood cells.

Homeostasis
A balanced condition that must be maintained in the body for health. Examples include fluid balance, chemical balance, glucose balance, and body temperature.

Hormone
A chemical messenger produced by one type of cell that travels through the bloodstream to change the actions of a different type of cell.

Hyperbaric Oxygen Therapy
Breathing pure oxygen in while in a pressurized chamber in order to increase the amount of oxygen in the blood and promote wound healing. This therapy is sometimes used to heal persistent diabetic ulcers. It is also used to treat decompression sickness (the bends) in scuba divers.

Hyperglycemia
An abnormally high level of glucose in the blood. It usually results from inadequate insulin to cover the amount of carbohydrates eaten. Hyperglycemia is a sign of all types of diabetes, and extreme hyperglycemia can result in diabetic ketoacidosis and death.

Hypoglycemia
An abnormally low level of glucose in the blood. Hypoglycemia can cause irregular heartbeat, confusion, seizures, loss of consciousness, and death. In diabetics, it usually results from a poor match between the amount of insulin and the amount of carbohydrates eaten.

Incretins
A group of hormones made in the small intestine and released during a meal that help trigger the release of insulin from beta cells and thus lower blood glucose levels.

Insulin Analog
An altered form of natural insulin that is made in a laboratory. Insulin analogs do not occur in nature, but they are similar enough to natural insulin to be used by the body. By making small changes in the insulin molecule, the peak effectiveness of an insulin analog and the length of time it is effective can be altered for better glycemic control. This has resulted in a variety of insulins analogs with different properties.

Insulin Resistance
The decreased sensitivity of cells to insulin. This makes it difficult for glucose to enter cells, where it is needed for energy, so blood glucose levels rise.

Islets of Langerhans
Most of the pancreas produces digestive enzymes. The islets of Langerhans, also called pancreatic islets, are clumps of cells embedded in the pancreas that produce glucose-regulating hormones. Insulin-producing beta cells and glucagon-producing alpha cells are the most common types of islet cells.

Juvenile Diabetes
An older name for type 1 diabetes that is no longer used.

Ketones
Chemicals that result from the breakdown of fat for energy when not enough glucose is available. Ketones make the blood more acidic and, if not treated, can result in diabetic ketoacidosis.

Oral Glucose Tolerance Test (OGTT)
A blood test used to screen for type 2 diabetes or gestational diabetes but not type 1 diabetes. It measures how easily glucose enters cells.

Placebo
A harmless substance given to some volunteers during a clinical trial so that their responses can be compared to volunteers who are given the trial drug.

Podiatrist
A doctor who specializes in treating foot problems.

Prediabetes
A condition in which blood glucose levels are higher than normal but not high enough to diagnose diabetes. The condition often progresses to diabetes, but, in many cases, can be reversed through diet and lifestyle changes.

Subcutaneous
Under the skin but above the muscle. This is the level at which insulin should be injected.

Triglycerides
Fats in the blood that can contribute to the development of arteriosclerosis.

Directory of Resources

Academy of Nutrition and Dietetics
120 S. Riverside Plaza, Suite 2190
Chicago, IL 60606-6995
1-312-899-0040
1-800-877-1600
https://www.eatright.org

American Association of Diabetes Educators
200 W. Madison Street, Suite 800
Chicago, IL 60606
1-800-338-3633
https://www.diabeteseducator.org

American Diabetes Association
2541 Crystal Drive, Suite 900
Alexandria, VA 22202
1-800-DIABETES (1-800-342-2383)
https://www.diabetes.org

Beyond Type 1
1001 Laurel Street, Suite B
San Carlos, CA 94070
650-924-5959
https://beyondtype1.org
Information in both English and Spanish

Diabetes at School (Canada)
Canadian Paediatric Society
100-2305 St. Laurent Boulevard
Ottawa, ON Canada K1G 4J8
613-526-9397
Fax: 613-526-3332
https://www.diabetesatschool.ca/schools/schools

Diabetes Canada
1400-522 University Avenue
Toronto, ON Canada M5G 2R5
416-363-3373
1-800-226-8464
Fax: 514 259-9286
https://www.diabetes.ca

Diabetes Québec
3750 Cremazie Boulevard, Suite 500
Montréal QC Canada H2A 1B6
514-259-3422
1-800-361-3504
Fax: 514 259-9286
https://www.diabete.qc.ca
Information and live chat in French and English

Diabetes Research Institute Foundation
200 S. Park Road, Suite 100
Hollywood, FL 33021
954-964-4040
800-321-3437
Fax: 954-964-7036
https://www.diabetesresearch.org

Dogs4Diabetics
1647 Willow Pass Road #157
Concord, CA 94520
925-246-5785
https://dogs4diabetics.com

European Foundation for the Study of Diabetes
Rheindorfer Weg 3
40591 Düsseldorf
Germany

+49-211-758-469-0
Fax: +49-211-758-469-29
http://www.europeandiabetesfoundation.org

InDependent Diabetes Trust
PO Box 294
Northampton, NN1 4XS
United Kingdom
01144 1604 622837
Fax: 01144 1604 622838
https://www.iddt.org

International Diabetes Foundation
166 Chaussee de La Hulpe
B-1170 Brussels, Belgium
+32-2-538-55-11
Fax +32-2-538-51-14
https://www.diabetesatlas.org

International Society for Pediatric and Adolescent Diabetes (ISPAD)
Kurfustendamn 71
10709 Berlin, Germany
+49 (0)30 24603-210
Fax: +49 (0)30 24603-200
https://www.ispad.org

Joslin Diabetes Center
A Harvard Medical School Affiliate
One Joslin Place
Boston, MA 02215
617-309-2400
https://www.joslin.org

Juvenile Diabetes Research Foundation
26 Broadway, 14th Floor
New York, NY 10004
1-800-533-CURE (2873)
Fax: 1-212-785-9595
https://www.jdrf.org

National Diabetes Services Scheme
Diabetes Australia
https://www.ndss.com.au

National Institute of Diabetes and Digestive and Kidney Diseases Health
Information Center
9000 Rockville Plaza
Bethesda, MD 20892
1-800-860-8747
TTY: 1-866-569-1162
https://www.niddk.nih.gov/health-information/diabetes

United States Centers for Disease Control and Prevention (CDC)
1600 Clifton Road
Atlanta, GA 30333
1-404-639-3534
1-800-CDC-INFO (1-800-232-4636)
TTY: 888-232-6348
https://www.cdc.gov

Bibliography

Alcorn, Ted. "The Strange Marketplace for Diabetic Test Strips." *New York Times*. January 14, 2019. Accessed November 6, 2019. https://www.nytimes.com/2019/01/14/health/diabetes-test-strips-resale.html.

Aleppo, Grazia. "Gestational Diabetes: What You Should Know." Endocrine Web. August 3, 2018. Accessed November 6, 2019. https://www.endocrineweb.com/conditions/gestational-diabetes/gestational-diabetes.

Ali, Naheed. *Diabetes and You: A Comprehensive Holistic Approach*. Lanham, MD: Rowman and Littlefield, 2011.

American College of Obstetricians and Gynecologists. "Pregnancy FAQ: Gestational Diabetes." November 2017. Accessed November 6, 2019. https://www.acog.org/Patients/FAQs/Gestational-Diabetes?

American Diabetes Association. "Diabetes and Driving." *Diabetes Care* 37, suppl. 1 (January 2014): S97–S108. Accessed November 6, 2019. https://care.diabetesjournals.org/content/37/Supplement_1/S97.

American Diabetes Association. "Insulin and Other Injectables." Undated. Accessed August 27, 2018. http://www.diabetes.org/living-with-diabetes/treatment-and-care/medication/insulin.

American Diabetes Association. *Managing Type 2 Diabetes for Dummies*. Hoboken, NJ: John Wiley and Sons, 2018.

Barnes-Svarney, Patricia, and Thomas E. Svarney. *The Handy Diabetes Answer Book*. Detroit, MI: Visible Ink, 2018.

Bautman, Vechi. "Diabetic Nephropathy." Medscape. October 9, 2019. Accessed November 6, 2019. https://emedicine.medscape.com/article/238946-overview.

Bellenir, Karen, ed. *Diabetes Information for Teens*, 2nd ed. Detroit, MI: Omnigraphics, 2012.

Belluz, Julia. "The Absurdly High Cost of Insulin, Explained." *Vox*. May 24, 2019. Accessed November 6, 2019. https://www.vox.com/2019/4/3/18293950/why-is-insulin-so-expensive.

Bhavsar, Abdhish. "Diabetic Retinopathy." Medscape. May 22, 2019. Accessed November 6, 2019. https://emedicine.medscape.com/article/1225122-overview.

Bliss, Michael. *The Discovery of Insulin*. Chicago IL: University of Chicago Press, 2007.

Boyd, Kierstan. "What Is Glaucoma?" American Academy of Ophthalmology. August 28, 2019. Accessed November 6, 2019. https://www.aao.org/eye-health/diseases/what-is-glaucoma.

Bryder, Linda, and Courtney Harper. "Commentary: More Than 'Tentative Opinions': Harry Himsworth and Defining Diabetes," *International Journal of Epidemiology* 42, no. 6 (December 2013): 1599–1600. Accessed November 6, 2019. https://academic.oup.com/ije/article/42/6/1599/742359.

Chaloner, Kim. *Diabetes and Me.* New York, NY: Hill and Wang, 2013.

Chiang, Jane L., M. Sue Kirkman, Lori M. B. Laffel, and Anne L. Peters. "Type 1 Diabetes Through the Life Span: A Position Statement of the American Diabetes Association." *Diabetes Care* 37, no. 7 (July 2014): 2034–2054. Accessed November 6, 2019. http://care.diabetesjournals.org/content/37/7/2034.

Colberg, Sheri R. *Diabetes and Keeping Fit for Dummies.* Hoboken, NJ: John Wiley and Sons, 2018.

Colberg, Sheri R. "Exercise and Type 2 Diabetes: The American College of Sports Medicine and the American Diabetes Association: Joint Position Statement." *Diabetes Care* 33, no. 12 (December 10, 2010): e147–e167. Accessed November 6, 2019. https://www.ncbi.nlm.nih.gov/pmc/articles/PMC2992225.

Cooper, Thea, and Arthur Ainsberg. *Breakthrough: Elisabeth Hughes, the Discovery of Insulin, and the Making of a Medical Miracle.* New York, NY: St Martin's Press, 2010.

Cornerstones4Care. "Playing Competitive Sports." September 2016. Accessed November 6, 2019. https://type1.cornerstones4care.com/being-active/growing-up-with-diabetes/playing-competitive-sports.html.

Cybersecurity and Infrastructure Security Agency. "ICS Medical Advisory (ICSMA-19-178-01): Medtronic MiniMed 508 and Paradigm Series Insulin Pumps." June 27, 2019. Accessed January 22, 2020. https://www.us-cert.gov/ics/advisories/icsma-19-178-01

Dagogo-Jack, Sam. *Diabetes Risks from Prescription and Nonprescription Drugs.* Alexandria, VA: American Diabetes Association, 2016.

Daneman, Denis, Shaun Barrett, and Jennifer Harrington. *When a Child Has Diabetes*, 4th ed. Toronto, Canada: Robert Rose, Inc., 2018.

Diabetes Australia. "Diabetes and Pregnancy." Undated. Accessed November 6, 2019. https://www.ndss.com.au/about-diabetes/pregnancy.

Diabetes.co.uk "Infertility in Men." Undated. Accessed November 6, 2019. https://www.diabetes.co.uk/pregnancy-complications/infertility-in-men.html.

Diabetic Council. "The History of Diabetes." The DiabeticCouncil.com. March 6, 2018. Accessed November 6, 2019. https://www.thediabetescouncil.com/the-history-of-diabetes.

Dinerstein, Chuck. "'Bionic Pancreas' Begins Clinical Trials." American Council on Health and Science. August 29, 2018. Accessed November 6, 2019. https://www.acsh.org/news/2018/08/29/bionic-pancreas-begins-clinical-trials-13248.

Dougherty, Jennifer P. "The Experience of Siblings of Children with Type 1 Diabetes." *Pediatric Nursing* 41, no. 6 (November–December 2015): 279–282.

Felman, Adam. "What Are Insulin Pens and How Do We Use Them?" Medical News Today. March 27, 2019. Accessed November 6, 2019. https://www.medicalnewstoday.com/articles/316607.php.

Fernández, Clara R. "The Future of Diabetes Treatment: Is a Cure Possible?" LabioTech. July 15, 2019. Accessed November 6, 2019. https://www.labiotech.eu/features/diabetes-treatment-cure-review.

Filippi, Christophe M., and Matthias G. von Herrath. "Viral Triggers for Type 1 Diabetes: Pros and Cons." *Diabetes* 57, no. 11 (November 2008): 2863–2871. Accessed November 6, 2019. https://www.ncbi.nlm.nih.gov/pmc/articles/PMC2570378.

Fisher, Lawrence. "Family Relationships and Diabetes Care During the Adult Years." *Diabetes Spectrum* 19, no. 2 (April 2006): 71–74. Accessed November 6, 2019. https://spectrum.diabetesjournals.org/content/19/2/71.

Ford-Martin, Paula. *The Everything Guide to Managing Type 2 Diabetes.* Avon, MA: Adams Media, 2013.

Gentile, Julie M. "Type 1 Diabetes Slideshow." Endocrine Web. 2019. Accessed November 6, 2019. https://www.endocrineweb.com/conditions/type-1-diabetes/managing-type-1-diabetes.

Gordon, Serena. "Pot Use Tied to Serious Diabetes Complication." WebMD. November 4, 2018. Accessed November 5, 2019. https://www.webmd.com/diabetes/news/20181108/pot-use-tied-to-serious-diabetes-complication#1.

Hamdy, Osama. "Diabetic Ketoacidosis." Medscape. May 31, 2019. Accessed November 6, 2019. https://emedicine.medscape.com/article/118361-overview.

Hauser, Christine. "Utah Family Sues after Son with Diabetes Is Kept from School." *New York Times.* June 29, 2019. Accessed November 6, 2019. https://www.nytimes.com/2019/06/29/us/utah-diabetes-school-lawsuit.html.

Helgeson, Vicki S., Dorothy Becker, Oscar Escobar, and Linda Siminerio. "Families with Children with Diabetes: Implications of Parent Stress and Child Health." *Journal of Pediatric Psychology* 37, no. 4 (May 2012): 467–478. Accessed November 6, 2019. https://academic.oup.com/jpepsy/article/37/4/467/894390.

Hess-Fischl, Amy. "Hyperglycemia: When Your Blood Glucose Level Goes Too High." EndocrineWeb. September 7, 2018. Accessed November 6, 2019. https://www.endocrineweb.com/conditions/hyperglycemia/hyperglycemia-when-your-blood-glucose-level-goes-too-high.

Hess-Fischl, Amy. "Hypoglycemia Overview: What Happens When Your Blood Glucose Level Drops Too Low." EndocrineWeb. September 7, 2018. Accessed November 6, 2019. https://www.endocrineweb.com/conditions/hypoglycemia/hypoglycemia-overview.

Hess-Fischl, Amy. "Prediabetes: How to Prevent Prediabetes from Becoming Type 2 Diabetes." EndocrineWeb. July 6, 2018. Accessed January 22, 2020. https://www.endocrineweb.com/conditions/pre-diabetes/pre-diabetes.

Home, Philip. "Controversies for Glucose Control Targets in Type 2 Diabetes: Exposing the Common Ground." *Diabetes Care* 42, no. 9 (September 2019): 1615–1623. Accessed September 30, 2019. https://care.diabetesjournals.org/content/42/9/1615.

Idlebrook, Craig. "Class-Action Lawsuit against Insulin Companies Clears Legal Hurdle." T1D Exchange Glu. April 24, 2019. Accessed November 6, 2019. https://myglu.org/articles/class-action-lawsuit-against-insulin-companies-clears-legal-hurdle.

Jensen, Jørgen, Per Inge Rustad, Anders Jensen Kolnes, and Yu-Chiang La. "The Role of Skeletal Muscle Glycogen Breakdown for Regulation of Insulin Sensitivity by Exercise." *Frontiers in Physiology* 2 (December 30, 2011): 112. Accessed November 6, 2019. https://www.frontiersin.org/articles/10.3389/fphys.2011.00112/full.

Juvenile Diabetes Research Foundation. "Teen Toolkit." 2013. Accessed November 6, 2019. https://www.jdrf.org/wp-content/uploads/2013/10/JDRFTEENTOOLKIT.pdf.

Kaufman, Francine. *Insulin Pumps and Continuous Glucose Monitoring: A User's Guide to Effective Diabetes Management*, 2nd ed. Arlington, VA: American Diabetes Association, 2017.

Khardori, Romesh. "Type 1 Diabetes Mellitus." Medscape. September 13, 2019. Accessed November 6, 2019. https://emedicine.medscape.com/article/117739-overview.

Khardori, Romesh. "Type 2 Diabetes Mellitus." Medscape. October 23, 2019. Accessed November 6, 2019. https://emedicine.medscape.com/article/117853-overview.

Krzewska, Aleksandra, and Iwona Ben-Skowronek. "Effect of Associated Autoimmune Diseases on Type 1 Diabetes Mellitus Incidence and Metabolic Control in Children and Adolescents." *BioMed Research International* 2016: 6219730. Epub July 20, 2016. Accessed November 6, 2019. https://www.ncbi.nlm.nih.gov/pmc/articles/PMC4971288.

Kühtreiber, Willem, Lisa Tran, Taesoo Kim, Michael Dybala, Brian Nguyen, Sara Plager, and Daniel Huang, et al. "Long-Term Reduction in Hyperglycemia in Advanced Type 1 Diabetes: The Value of Induced Aerobic Glycolysis with BCG Vaccinations." *npj Vaccines* 3, no. 23 (June 18, 2018). Accessed November 6, 2019. https://www.nature.com/articles/s41541-018-0062-8.

Lakhtakia, Ritu. "The History of Diabetes Mellitus." *Sultan Qaboos University Medical Journal* 13, no. 3 (August 2013): 368–370. Accessed November 6, 2019. https://www.ncbi.nlm.nih.gov/pmc/articles/PMC3749019.

Lamb, William H. "Pediatric Type 1 Diabetes Mellitus." Medscape. July 3, 2019. Accessed November 6, 2019. https://emedicine.medscape.com/article/919999-overview.

Lee, Benita. "How Much Does Insulin Cost?—Here's How 23 Brands Compare." Good Rx. August 23, 2019. Accessed November 6, 2019. https://www.goodrx.com/blog/how-much-does-insulin-cost-compare-brands.

Leonard, Jayne, "Can Marijuana Help People with Diabetes?" Medical News Today. March 27, 2019. Accessed November 6, 2019. https://www.medicalnewstoday.com/articles/316999.php.

Leontis, Lisa M. "Type 2 Diabetes: Key Facts." EndocrineWeb. 2019. Accessed November 6, 2019. https://www.endocrineweb.com/conditions/type-2-diabetes/type-2-diabetes-overview.

Manzu, Allan. "Why Were 'Starvation Diets' Promoted for Diabetes in the Pre-Insulin Period?" *Nutrition Journal* 10 (2010): 23. Accessed November 6, 2019. https://www.ncbi.nlm.nih.gov/pmc/articles/PMC3062586.

Mayo Clinic Staff. "Diabetic Ketoacidosis." Mayo Clinic. June 12, 2018. Accessed November 6, 2019. https://www.mayoclinic.org/diseases-conditions/diabetic-ketoacidosis/symptoms-causes/syc-20371551.

McMillen, Matt. "Is Bariatric Surgery Right for You?" *Diabetes Forecast*. May 2018. Accessed November 6, 2019. http://www.diabetesforecast.org/2018/03-may-jun/is-bariatric-surgery-right.html?loc=morefrom.

Mental Health America. "Diabetes and Mental Health." 2019. Accessed November 6, 2019. https://www.mentalhealthamerica.net/conditions /diabetes-and-mental-health.

Moore, Thomas R. "Diabetes Mellitus and Pregnancy." Medscape. April 11, 2018. Accessed November 6, 2019. https://emedicine.medscape .com/article/127547-overview.

Morstein, Mona. *Master Your Diabetes.* White River Junction, VT: Chelsea Green Publishing, 2017.

National Institute of Diabetes and Digestive and Kidney Diseases. "The A1c Test and Diabetes." April 2018. Accessed November 6, 2019. https://www.niddk.nih.gov/health-information/diabetes/overview /tests-diagnosis/a1c-test#affected.

National Institute of Diabetes and Digestive and Kidney Diseases. "Diabetic Kidney Disease." February 2017. Accessed November 6, 2019. https://www.niddk.nih.gov/health-information/diabetes/overview /preventing-problems/diabetic-kidney-disease.

National Institute of Diabetes and Digestive and Kidney Diseases. "Pancreatic Islet Transplantation." October 2018. Accessed November 6, 2019. https://www.niddk.nih.gov/health-information/diabetes/overview /insulin-medicines-treatments/pancreatic-islet-transplantation.

National Institute of Diabetes and Digestive and Kidney Diseases, "Preventing Diabetes Problems" Undated. Accessed November 6, 2019. https://www.niddk.nih.gov/health-information/diabetes/overview /preventing-problems.

Olatunbosun, Samuel. "Glucose Intolerance." Medscape. June 28, 2019. Accessed November 6, 2019. https://emedicine.medscape.com /article/119020-overview#a6.

Oleck, Jacob, Shahista Kassam, and Jennifer D. Goldman. "Commentary: Why Was Inhaled Insulin a Failure in the Market?" *Diabetes Spectrum* 29, no. 3 (August 2016): 180–184. Accessed November 6, 2019. https://spectrum.diabetesjournals.org/content/29/3/180.

Patel, Sonal J. "Gestational Diabetes Testing Protocol." Medscape. March 19, 2019. Accessed November 6, 2019. https://emedicine.medscape .com/article/2049380-overview.

Peters, Anne, and Lori Laffel, eds. *Type 1 Diabetes Sourcebook.* Arlington, VA: American Diabetes Association, 2018.

Pollreisz, Andreas, and Ursula Schmidt-Erfurth. "Diabetic Cataracts— Pathogenesis, Epidemiology and Treatment." *Journal of Ophthalmology* 2010, Article ID 60875. Accessed November 6, 2019. https:// www.hindawi.com/journals/joph/2010/608751.

Poretsky, Leonid. *Principles of Diabetes Mellitus.* New York, NY: Springer, 2017.

Quan, Dianna. "Diabetic Neuropathy." Medscape. July 23, 2019. Accessed November 6, 2019. https://emedicine.medscape.com/article/1170337 -overview.

Quianzon, Celeste, and Issam Cheikh. "History of Insulin." *Journal of Community Hospital Internal Medicine Perspectives* 2, no. 2 (2012). Published online July 16, 2012. Accessed November 6, 2019. https:// www.ncbi.nlm.nih.gov/pmc/articles/PMC3714061.

Richardson, Sarah J., and Noel G. Morgan. "Enteroviral Infection in the Pathogenesis of Type 1 Diabetes: New Insights for Therapeutic Intervention." *Current Opinion in Pharmacology* 43 (December 2018): 11–19. Accessed November 6, 2019. https://www.ncbi.nlm .nih.gov/pmc/articles/PMC6294842.

Sacks, David A., ed. *Diabetes and Pregnancy*. Alexandria, VA: American Diabetes Association, 2011.

Sanders, Lee J. "From Thebes to Toronto and the 21st Century: An Incredible Journey." *Diabetes Spectrum* 15, no. 1 (January 2002): 56–60. Accessed November 6, 2019. https://spectrum.diabetesjournals.org /content/15/1/56.

Scheiner, Gary, and Diane Herbert. *Diabetes—How to Help*. Alexandria, VA: American Diabetes Association, 2011.

Sherman, Irwin W. *Drugs That Changed the World*. Boca Raton, FL: CRC Press, 2016.

Shubrook, Jay, William Chen, and Alegria Lim. "Evidence for the Prevention of Type 2 Diabetes Mellitus." *Journal of the American Osteopathic Association* 118 (November 2018): 703–737. Accessed November 6, 2019. https://jaoa.org/article.aspx?articleid=271 2300.

Silve, Marta. "High Blood-Sugar Levels Seen to Affect How Blood Vessels Contract." *Diabetes News Journal*. January 20, 2016. Accessed November 6, 2019. https://diabetesnewsjournal.com/2016/01/20 /high-blood-sugar-levels-seen-affect-blood-vessels-contract.

Snouffer, Elizabeth. "What Is Diabetes Distress?" Beyond Type 1. Undated. Accessed November 6, 2019. https://beyondtype1.org/what-is -diabetes-distress.

Stanford Children's Health. "Diabetes and Pregnancy." 2019. Accessed November 6, 2019. https://www.stanfordchildrens.org/en/topic /default?id=diabetes-and-pregnancy-90-P02444.

Tabák, Adam, Christian Herder, Wolfgang Rathmann, Ericand J. Brunner, Mika Kivamaki. "Prediabetes: A High-risk State for Developing Diabetes." *Lancet* 379, no. 9833 (June 16, 2012): 2279–2290. Accessed November 6, 2019. https://www.ncbi.nlm.nih.gov/pmc /articles/PMC3891203.

Tanner, Courtney. "A Utah Family Is Suing after an Elementary School Blocked Their Diabetic Son from Going to Class." *Salt Lake Tribune.* June 27, 2019. Accessed November 6, 2019. https://www.sltrib .com/news/education/2019/06/26/utah-family-is-suing.

Tsai, Allison. "6 Tests to Determine Diabetes Type." *Diabetes Forecast.* September 2015. Accessed November 6, 2019. http://www .diabetesforecast.org/2015/sep-oct/tests-to-determine-diabetes .html.

United States Food and Drug Administration. "What Is the Pancreas? What Is an Artificial Pancreas Device System?" August 30, 2018. Accessed November 6, 2019. https://www.fda.gov/medical-devices /artificial-pancreas-device-system/what-pancreas-what-artificial -pancreas-device-system.

University of California, San Francisco. "Goals of Treatment." Diabetes Education Online. Undated. Accessed November 6, 2019. https:// dtc.ucsf.edu/types-of-diabetes/type1/treatment-of-type-1-diabetes /monitoring-diabetes/goals-of-treatment.

University of California, San Francisco. "Insulin Analogs." Diabetes Education Online. Undated. Accessed November 6, 2019. https://dtc .ucsf.edu/types-of-diabetes/type2/treatment-of-type-2-diabetes /medications-and-therapies/type-2-insulin-rx/types-of-insulin /insulin-analogs.

White, John R. "A Brief History of the Development of Diabetes Medications." *Diabetes Spectrum* 27, no. 2 (May 2014): 82–26. Accessed November 6, 2019. https://spectrum.diabetesjournals.org/content /27/2/82.full.

Wood, Jamie, and Anne Peters. *The Type 1 Diabetes Self-Care Manual.* Arlington, VA: American Diabetes Association, 2018.

Wooley, Elizabeth. "How Insulin Works in the Body: The Multiple Roles of This Vital Hormone." Very Well Health. October 30, 2019. Accessed November 6, 2019. https://www.verywellhealth.com/how-insulin -works-in-the-body-1087716.

Wu, Brian. "History of Diabetes: Past Treatments and New Discoveries." Medical News Today. April 29, 2019. Accessed November 6, 2019. https://www.medicalnewstoday.com/articles/317484.php.

Index

Page numbers followed by *t* indicate tables.

Acarbose, 73
Alcohol, 57–58, 114
Allen, Frederick, 16–17
Allen diet, 16–17, 23
Alpha cells, 3, 4, 5, 8, 35, 139
Alpha-glucosidase inhibitors, 73, 97
American Dental Association, 98
American Diabetes Association, 10, 36, 43, 45, 99, 109, 122, 131, 135
Americans with Disabilities Act, 109–110, 112, 113
Amylin, 5, 6
Amylin agonists, 75
Antibody testing, 48–49
A1c, 47, 48*t*, 51, 52*t*, 66, 71, 72, 73, 74, 112, 115, 123, 135–136, 139, 140–141
Athletes with diabetes, 34, 50
Athlete's foot, 92, 93
Athletics. *See* Sports participation
Autoimmunity, 1, 6, 31, 32, 34, 119–120, 122, 140
Autonomic neuropathy, 90

Banting, Frederick: death, 27; education, 17–18; and first insulin patient, 23–24; initial failures, 20–21; inspiration for insulin, 18; Nobel Prize, 26; relationship with Collip, 24–25; relationship with Macleod, 19, 21, 22–23, 24, 26
Bariatric surgery, 76, 126
Barron, Moses, 18
Basal insulin dose, 54, 65, 66
BCG vaccine, 140–141
Bernard, Claude, 15
Best, Charles, 20, 21, 22–25, 26, 27
Beta cells, 3, 4, 5–7, 8, 31–33, 35, 43, 48, 119, 123, 138, 139, 141
Biguanides, 31, 71–72
Bile acid sequestrants, 74
Birth control pills, 46, 100
Blood glucose monitoring, 58–59; with electromagnetic waves, 143
Blood glucose regulation: hormonal, 35–36; measuring, 2–6; values, 3*t*
Body Mass Index (BMI), 36, 45, 123
Bolus insulin dose, 54, 55, 56, 64–65
Bromocriptine, 75

Camps for diabetics, 109
Canagliflozin, 74
Candida albicans, 93, 98
Cannabinoids (CBD), 115
Carbohydrates, counting, 54–57
Caregivers: burnout, 101, 117; education of, 112–113
Cataracts, 87–88

Cellulitis, 93–94
Charcot's foot, 91, 93
Chevreul, Michel-Eugéne, 15
Clowes, George, 25–26
Cochran, Kyle, 50
Colesevelam, 74
Collip, James Bertram, 22, 25, 26, 27–28; Nobel Prize, 26; relationship with Banting, 24–25, 28
Complications: acute, 79–80; cardiovascular, 81–84; chronic, 80–81; eye, 84–88; feet, 90–93; gastrointestinal, 96–97; kidney, 95–96; liver, 97–98; nervous system, 88–90; oral, 98; of pregnancy, 101–103; psychological, 100–101, 115–117; sexual, 99–101, 114
Connaught Laboratory, 24, 25, 26
Continuous glucose monitors (CGMs), 60–61, 65
Coronary artery disease, 82–83
C-peptide protein, 48
Cullen, William, 14
Cutler, Jay, 40

Delta cells, 3, 6
Diabetes: in ancient times, 13–14; costs, 10–11, 130–132, 142; in 18th century, 14; in 19th century, 15; uncommon forms, 4, 34
Diabetes Autoimmune Study in the Young (DAISY), 122
Diabetes distress, 101
Diabetes insipidus, 14
Diabetes Medical Management Plan (DMMP), 110
Diabetic ketoacidosis (DKA), 7, 31, 32, 43, 44, 49–50, 59, 65, 119, 131
Diabetic kidney disease (DKD), 95–96
Diabetic macular edema, 73, 86–87
Diabetic retinopathy, 85–86, 87
Diagnostic tests. See Tests
Dietary supplements, 121, 126–127
Dipeptidyl-peptidase 4 (DPP-4) inhibitors, 74, 97
Dobson, Matthew, 14
Driving, 107, 114

Dudley, Chris, 50
Dulaglutide, 73
Dwarfism, 28, 51

Employment laws, 113
End stage renal disease (ESRD), 95–96
Endocrine cells, 3
Enteropathy, diabetic, 96–97
Epsilon cells, 3, 6
Erectile dysfunction (ED), 44, 90, 99
Erysipelas, 94
Erythrasma, 94
European Nicotinamide Diabetes Intervention Trial, 121
Exenatide, 73
Exercise. See Physical activity
Exocrine cells, 3

Family response to diagnosis, 101, 105, 107–109, 115–116
Fasting blood glucose, 3t, 38, 44, 46
Fatty liver, 97–98
Fehling, Hermann von, 15
504 plan, 109–110
Flesh-eating disease, 94
Focal neuropathy, 90

Gamma cells, 6
Gastroesophageal reflux disease, 97
Gastroparesis, 96
Genentech, Inc., 29
Gestational diabetes, 1, 9–10, 37–39, 44, 46–47, 76–77, 86, 101–103, 119, 125, 127
Glaucoma, 87
Glimepiride, 72
Glipizide, 72
Glitazones. See Thiazolidinediones
Glucagon, 5, 35–36, 75, 110, 113, 139
Glucagon-like peptide-1 agonists, 73–74
Glucose: chemical composition, 2; foods high in, 2, 4
Glucose meters, 59, 61
Glucose monitoring. See Blood glucose monitoring

Glucose regulation. *See* Blood glucose regulation
Glyburide, 72
Glycated hemoglobin test. *See* A1c
Goeddel, David, 29

Hall, Gary, Jr., 50
Hammertoe, 91
Heartburn, 97
Himsworth, Sir Harold Percival, 28
Homeostasis, 2, 32, 35, 75
Hughes, Charles Evans, 17
Hughes, Elizabeth, 17, 26–27
Hyperglycemia, 2, 6, 10, 31, 35, 36, 42, 49, 66, 76–77
Hyperosmolar hyperglycemic state, 79–80
Hypoglycemia, 2, 51–52, 61, 72, 75, 90, 101, 127; and alcohol, 57–58, 114; in newborns, 39, 102
Hypothalamus, 5, 6, 75

Impetigo, 94
Incretins, 73, 74
Infections, 44, 74, 92–94, 100
Insulin: analogs, 20–30, 53–54, 55*t*; from animals, 28–29, 52, 53, 130; brands, 55*t*; cost, 26, 129–134; experimental, 142; function, 4–5; inhaled, 54, 55*t*, 66; Nobel Prize, 26; patent, 24–25, 130, 132; storage requirements, 63–64; synthetic, 28–29, 53, 55*t*, 130; syringe injection, 62–63
Insulin pens, 63–64
Insulin politics, 129, 131, 134
Insulin pumps, 64–66
Insulin resistance, 8, 28, 35, 36, 37, 38, 39, 69, 72, 77, 102, 123, 142
insulin-to-carbohydrate ratio (I:C), 55–56
Intermediate hyperglycemia. *See* Prediabetes
Islet cell transplantation, 138–139
Isletin, 20, 25
Islets of Langerhans. *See* Pancreatic islets

Jock itch, 93
Juvenile diabetes. *See* Type 1

Ketones, 7, 31, 32, 43, 49; testing, 58, 61–63

Laguesse, Gustave-Édouard, 15
Lancets, 60
Langerhans, Paul, 15
Latent autoimmune diabetes in adults (LADA), 1, 34
Laws: federal, 109–110, 112, 113; school district, 111; state, 110–111, 134
Lixisenatide, 73

Macleod, John James Rickard, 18, 19; death, 17; Nobel Prize, 26; relationship with Banting, 19, 21, 22–23, 24, 26
Marijuana, 114–115
Meglitinide derivatives, 72
Menstrual cycle, 100
Mering, Joseph von, 15, 19
Metformin, 30, 71–72, 77, 125–126
Microbiome modification, 141–142
Miglitol, 73
Minkowski, Oskar, 15, 19

National Athletic Trainers' Association, 112
Necrotizing fasciitis, 94
Neuropathies, 88–90
Nonalcoholic fatty liver disease (NAFLD), 97
Nonalcoholic steatohepatitis (NASH), 98
Nordisk Insulin Laboratory. *See* Novo Nordisk
Novo Nordisk, 26, 28, 53, 63, 131, 133, 142

Obesity and type 2, 6, 36, 69, 81, 97, 99, 123, 134
Oral contraceptives, 46, 100
Oral glucose tolerance test (OGTT), 45–47

Pancreas, 3, 4, 6, 29, 48, 72, 73, 102, 123; animal, 7, 15–16, 20, 22, 26, 53; "artificial," 137–138
Pancreatic islets, 3, 5–6, 15, 18, 33
Parents response to diagnosis, 100, 106–107
Patents, 24–25, 130, 132
Peripheral artery disease (PAD), 83–84
Peripheral diabetic neuropathy, 89
Peyronie's disease, 99
pH, 31, 32
Pharmacy benefit managers, 132–133
Physiatric Institute, 17. *See also* Allen, Frederick
Physical activity recommendations, 36–37
Pioglitazone, 72
Polycystic ovary syndrome (PCOS), 37, 39, 100
Post traumatic stress syndrome (PTSD), 106
PP cells, 6
Prediabetes, 1, 2, 3*t*, 9, 38, 43, 46, 47, 67, 69, 71, 122–124, 126–127, 141
Pregnancy, 103
Prognosis, 11, 103–104
Protamine zinc insulin (PZI), 28
Proximal neuropathy, 89

Random glucose test, 46
Rehabilitation Act, 109, 113
Repaglinide, 72
Retinopathy, 85–86, 87
Ringworm, 93
Rosiglitazone, 72

Sanofi, 53, 131, 133
School accommodations, 109–122
Semaglutide, 73
Service dogs, 127–128
Sotomayor, Sonia, 50
Sports participation, 50, 54, 110, 112
Starvation diet. *See* Allen diet

Statistics, 11, 34, 36, 38, 39, 103, 104
Stroke, 81, 83
Sulfonylureas, 71, 72, 74, 77
Support groups, 101, 113

Tests, diagnostic, 45–49
Test strips, 59, 61
Thiazolidinediones (TZDs), 71, 72–73, 100
Thompson, Leonard, 23–24
Thrush, 98
Tinea capitis, 93
Tinea corporis, 93
Tinea curis, 93
Tinea pedis, 92, 93
Travel precautions, 71, 113–114
Trial to Reduce Diabetes in the Genetically At-Risk (TRIGR), 120–121
Type 1 diabetes: causes, 6, 31–33; diagnosis, 3*t*, 14, 15, 46–49; management goals, 51, 52*t*; prevention studies, 120–122; risk factors, 7, 32–34; statistics, 7, 34, 104; stress, 106–109; symptoms, 41–43
Type 2 diabetes: causes, 35–36; diagnosis, 3*t*, 46–49; insulin use, 75–76; management, 66, 67–69, 70–80; prevention studies, 124–127; risk factors, 8, 35–38

University of Toronto, 17, 18, 19, 22, 24, 25, 27, 130

Vaccine Bacille Calmette-Guérin (BCG), 140–141

Weight loss drugs, 126
World Diabetes Day, 27, 105

Yeast, 29, 130, 133; infection, 44, 74, 93, 100

About the Author

Tish Davidson, AM, is a medical writer specializing in making technical information accessible to a general readership. Her previous books include *Fluids and Electrolytes*; *Vaccines: History, Science, and Issues*; and *The Vaccine Debate*. Davidson holds membership in the American Medical Writers Association and the American Society of Journalists and Authors.